The Beauty Brief

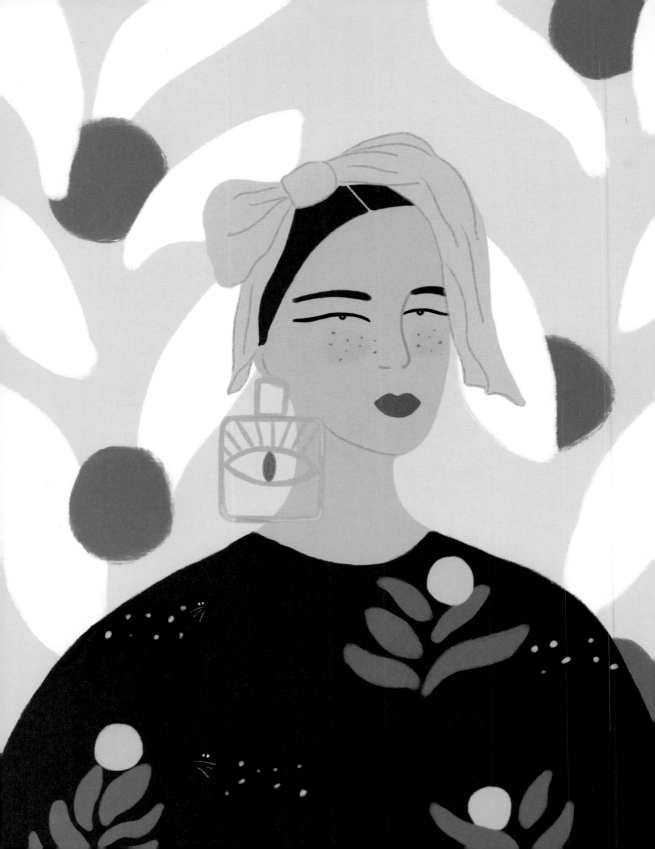

Katie Service

The Beauty Brief

An Insider's Guide to Skincare

Illustrations by
Constanza Goeppinger

Contents

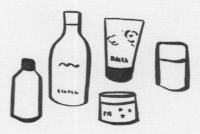

Skin is In

The science and secrets
behind skincare and the
beauty industry.
Think smarter; look better.

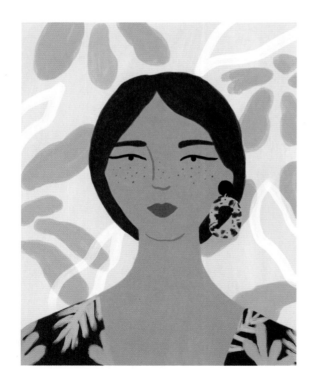

Welcome to your gloriously glossy glossary of skincare terminology. At your fingertips is a compendium of "skinformation" from me, a beauty editor, to you, designed to arm you with a greater knowledge about what exactly you are picking off the shelves. Take this book with you shopping, or keep it next to your laptop; consume it all at once, or feel free to dip in and out.

People regularly ask me the question, "Which moisturizer is better, X or Y?" My answer is always the same: "Have you checked what they're made from?" To which the response is nearly always: "No." And to be honest, I don't blame them for not bothering to check. Skincare ingredient lists – or "INCIs", as we call them in the biz (see p. 168) – are not particularly user-friendly. They are usually long, winding compilations of impenetrable science that are nigh-on impossible to understand, and who has the time? If it wasn't my job, I wouldn't either; I would be happy just to buy that moisturizer and believe all the wonderful promises on its label about looking younger, richer and more fabulous.

And that's how I know there are a lot of people out there who are just bluffing their way through skincare, taking the marketing jargon on the front as a given and totally ignoring the small print on the back because, hey, life is too short. And, on the whole, skincare brands aren't trying to pull the wool over your eyes – it's just that it's a competitive industry, and brands will go to great lengths to convince you to shop with them.

And when I say competitive, I mean *really* competitive. Bolstered by trends for "lockdown" skincare regimes, DIY beauty and post-pandemic wellbeing, recent times have seen a surge in the skincare industry; as a global market, it's predicted to be worth $190 billion by 2025. Meanwhile, the science behind the technologies and ingredients just gets better and better: skincare is now an arena for Nobel Laureate chemists, NASA scientists and stem-cell specialists. Meaning that, as a customer,

you need to get geeky. Knowing your skincare from the inside out has never been so important.

Another thing I've learned is that skincare isn't one size fits all. That a moisturizer you loved five years ago and have habitually used daily may not work the same wonders as it once did. That what works for Caucasian skin may not do the same thing for black skin or Asian skin.

I am not a scientist, and this is not a textbook, but I am quite obsessed with skincare. I frequently pull pots of moisturizer out of my coat pocket when I reach for my wallet while I'm out and about. I enjoy regular facials, peels, tweaks and lifts, and my bathroom cabinet is a sight to behold. As a beauty editor I also have access to some of the best dermatologists, facialists and formulators in the world, many of whose tips and advice I have shared in this book. But in the end I am just a normal woman on the hunt for answers and a less exhausted complexion.

Whatever your skin concerns – wrinkles, breakouts or other – I hope that this little book of definitions, tips and explanations can demystify the beauty industry and help you ask the right questions and find the answers you're looking for, whether these concern cost, care for the environment, ethics, or simply whether a product really works.

To help you navigate, some handy symbols are used throughout the book:

 An ingredient or product you'll find in my bathroom

 An ingredient or product that has a positive impact on the world (environmentally friendly, vegan, vegan-friendly, sustainable, fair trade, or otherwise impacting the planet positively)

 An ingredient or product to avoid

 The cost of a treatment or procedure

"Your body is so clever. If we could unzip our skin, we would unfold like a universe. That's how you need to look at it."

Nichola Joss, Facialist

"Beauty is such a nice way of examining the world."

Ateh Jewel, Beauty Journalist

"Good skincare is so important to incredible makeup. Since the beginning of my career I have always believed that the key to a beautiful painting lies in creating a beautiful canvas, and that taking care of your skin and having a good everyday skincare routine is essential. The key to magic skin is all about looking after and maintaining the best skin of your life. I love sharing my tips and tricks for skincare as much as I do for makeup."

Charlotte Tilbury, Makeup Artist
and Brand Founder

The
Big Issues

Your beauty industry
101 - the conversations
worth listening to.

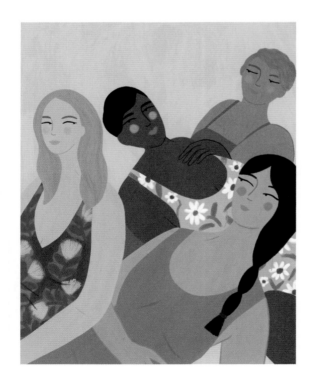

We live in an age when we are more interested than ever in the chemicals we interact with on a daily basis. We google them, we tweet about them, we read about them in newspapers, and we spend hours watching skincare tutorials and trawling through product reviews on Instagram.

That's what I love about beauty. Beyond its superficial trappings of lipstick and hairspray, it has a relevance in so many people's lives and so many social contexts. It also has a penchant for the political: just look at the way that brands like MAC and The Body Shop tap into bigger conversations on topics such as gender equality, animal rights, cultural appropriation and sustainability. It's never simply skin-deep.

However, the beauty industry has not always been known for landing on the right side of headline issues. There's still a vast misrepresentation in beauty when it comes to diversity, be that models' ethnicity, age or physical ability. The reality of skincare as deeply personalized is not yet being reflected in the way it's being sold to us. In addition, the industry is one that continues to use an incomprehensibly huge amount of plastic; we are quite literally filling the oceans with empty compacts and shampoo bottles. It's also an industry that has been guilty of promoting impossible standards and fuelling an unnerving trend for surgery and injectables in young people.

But, as with any industry, it has its superheroes, change-makers and pioneers, all striving to create a better, happier beauty world and to make us all feel more comfortable in our skin. Examples of beauty doing good include: Marcia Kilgore, whose bodycare line Soaper Duper supports WaterAid and offers formulations that can be washed down the plughole with a clean conscience; Mark Constantine, the CEO of Lush, which is selling foundation sticks coated in wax instead of plastic; the duo behind La Bouche Rouge, which offers one vegan leather refillable lipstick case, which you keep for life;

the British Beauty Council, set up by businesswoman Millie Kendall MBE to champion the rights of those working within the UK beauty industry, which worked tirelessly to get government clarification on how hairdressers, beauticians and manicurists could return safely to work post-COVID-19; Beauty Banks, a non-profit charity set up by journalist Sali Hughes and PR Jo Jones, to which individuals and brands can donate products that are then given to people in need; and Haircuts4Homeless, a UK community organization that provides shaves, haircuts and a dose of self-worth to people living on the streets.

As a beauty editor, I see the best and the worst in this complex industry, and so it's my job to help you navigate the ethics of the products you're browsing, as well as the contents. Here are some of the conversations I think are worth listening to (and even joining in with).

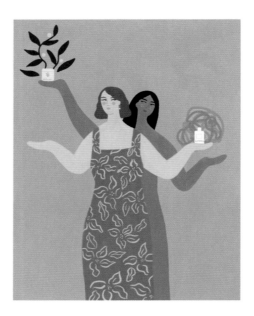

Naturals vs. Synthetics

Let's clear one thing up: all ingredients that find their way into beauty products are chemicals. Chemicals are simply substances that consist of matter. The term "chemical" can therefore mean any liquid, solid or gas, and encompasses natural or synthetic, made from one pure element or mixed as a compound or solution. So, to say that a face cream is "chemical-free" (and as a beauty editor I see this a lot from brands who are trying to jump on the naturals bandwagon) is, in fact, mismarketing. You need to know that when brands are pushing "chemical-free" formulas, they are just using scare tactics to trick you into buying their product.

What you really want to pay attention to is the level of synthetics vs. the level of naturals within your creams and lotions. It's impossible to say that all synthetics are bad for you and all naturals are good for you – there are plenty of synthetic chemicals that will do you no harm, and plenty of natural chemicals that could harm you. Each ingredient needs to be assessed on a case-by-case basis. The "clean beauty" movement would have you living, commune-style, away from all synthetics, but in contrast many dermatologists will warn you off 100% natural formulas, which may have a higher risk of causing allergic reactions and carrying bacteria. I can see both sides but given that, according to the Huffington Post, the average woman exposes her skin to 515 synthetic chemicals every day, I am inclined to think that keeping the synthetic count down in your cosmetics is an OK idea.

In skincare I would generally opt for natural ingredients, except under the following circumstances:

- The natural alternative is less effective and jeopardizes the health of your skin or the longevity of the product. This is relevant in the case of sunscreens and preservatives, where doing without synthetics could allow untold UV damage to your skin or cause an allergic reaction if the product was to go off.

- The natural alternative is likely to cause a reaction. Some natural ingredients are extremely reactive or sensitizing. Essential oils, for example, are 100% natural but too strong for many people's skin.

- The natural alternative is bad for the planet. This includes ingredients such as palm oil, which destroys the rainforest in its production, or almond oil from California, which needs an enormous amount of water to grow the almonds and is the cause of some serious droughts in the state.

So, how can you tell the natural percentage of a product? Unfortunately, you have to trust a brand to communicate with you honestly. If the "percentage natural" isn't stated on the packaging, then do your research and check out the company website. You could drop them an email to ask, or even send a tweet. It's easy to feel that you can't speak to the people behind your pot of skincare, but often they are very happy to hear from you.

Note that "clean beauty" is a made-up marketing term which implies that the product has reduced "nasties" – namely, synthetics, plastics, chemicals that are harmful to the skin or environment, and animal by-products. There is no one governing body over what makes something clean or natural. Providing a product contains a natural ingredient, it can claim to be natural to some extent, so there is a lot of uncertainty from the consumer standpoint. Independent governing bodies exist that monitor organic ingredients, such as Ecocert, which is one of the largest organic regulatory boards in the world, but brands have to apply to have the Ecocert stamp on their packaging, so it isn't omnipresent (see p. 166 for guidance on the symbols and other elements on the back of packaging, which can help you identify the naturalness of your cosmetics).

If you have decided you want to squeeze a little more natural beauty in your life but you really don't want to have to change your lifestyle dramatically or start churning up body butters in your kitchen, then follow these simple hacks:

◇ There are no redeeming features to face wipes (most of them being non-biodegradable, consisting of synthetic formulas embedded in synthetic poly-fibres), but you can buy washable eye makeup remover pads made of linen and flannel from zero-waste outlets. You won't notice the difference, but your skin and the planet will.

◇ Instead of using synthetic makeup removers, you can clean your makeup off with a natural oil. You can use coconut oil, straight from the tub in the fridge, or, if that's a little too eco for you, the natural brand Votary sells a brilliant cleansing oil, a blend of rose, geranium and apricot.

◇ Natural shower gels are another easy swap that your household will barely notice. Green People and Burt's Bees are two trustworthy brands that cost no more than majority-synthetics brands such as Radox or Molton Brown.

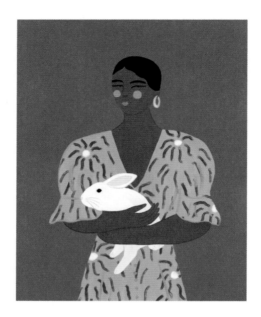

Vegan and Cruelty-Free

When the first few vegan beauty products started to land on my desk, I thought: this will never catch on. How wrong I was. Vegan beauty is booming, Boots recorded a 56% increase in vegan-related searches online in 2019. We know that Millennials care considerably about positive consuming, and this is what is finally starting to influence the way in which skincare brands formulate. Great news if you're a lab rat...

Animal welfare is important to this "Green Generation", which is why most brands who have launched in recent years are likely to position themselves as firmly anti-animal testing, cruelty-free, and either vegan or at least "vegan-friendly".

This is also because many of these brands, such as Westman Atelier, Hourglass, Milk Makeup and Drunk Elephant, are children of internet communities, where a huge emphasis is placed on transparency and positive core brand values. "Authenticity" has become a buzzword among these communities (and the brands that are trying to market to them).

The terminology that surrounds vegan beauty is a little confusing, though, so here are some handy definitions:

Vegan: A product that contains no ingredients that are derived from animals. That means no animal by-products either, such as beeswax, gelatin or ambergris (the sticky stuff found in whale stomachs that is harvested from beaches and considered an aphrodisiac in perfumery).

Vegan-friendly: A slightly looser term, which may be a brand's way of saying that no ingredients are sourced directly from animals, but – and this is a big but – the products may be made in the same factory as non-vegan cosmetics, or they may contain ingredients that are animal by-products, i.e. ingredients that are created by animals such as beeswax or egg white but don't technically harm the animal in their extraction.

"I always find vegan beauty products misleading. Surprisingly to most, vegan formulations aren't by default natural. Synthetic ingredients are often used in place of natural ingredients in order to obtain the vegan stamp. I feel, if you are going as far as to be so considerate of animal by-products on your skin, these shouldn't be substituted with non-natural synthetic ingredients that could potentially cause more harm than good."

Haley Bloom Fitzpatrick,
New Product Developer

Cruelty-free: A label which implies that no animal testing has been entered into. It's worth noting that any brand that imports into China currently has, by Chinese law, to submit their products to Chinese animal testing. The brand may not do this themselves, but by agreeing to sell in China they are condoning animal testing in that region. That said, the younger generation of Chinese consumers is waking up to the global mindset when it comes to animal testing, and the laws here – and elsewhere – are on their way to being reformed in the future.

Vegan Society Approved: If a product is marked with a Vegan Society logo, it means that no animal was involved or harmed in the making of the product.

Bunny logos: Stamps of approval from PETA (People for the Ethical Treatment of Animals), which confirm that neither animal testing nor animal cruelty were involved in the making of the product (see p. 167). PETA also have a handy list of non-vegan, animal-derived ingredients on their website if you want to double-check.

As with food, many beauty fans (myself included) aren't clean-cut when it comes to vegan beauty. They like the idea of it, but can't commit entirely. I am all for vegan beauty and I am firmly against animal testing, but there are certain ingredients I would still consider worth consuming.

- Animal by-products such as beeswax, ambergris and lanolin (which is extracted from sheep's wool). I personally don't have a problem with consuming ingredients that are harvested responsibly and that don't harm animals.

- Hyaluronic acid. This wonder moisturizer can be obtained from bioferments of plants and can therefore be 100% vegan, but this is not always the case. In China it's often grown on bacteria, and in Europe it can be extracted from animal parts such as rooster combs. I'm a sucker for the hydration that hyaluronic acid provides my skin; I suppose this is my skincare version of a free-pass Big Mac...

- Retinol (vitamin A). This is one of the most proven anti-ageing skincare ingredients, but it can be derived from animals, and unfortunately it's often hard to discover from a label whether the product uses retinol that's plant- or animal-derived. I'll admit I often turn a blind eye...

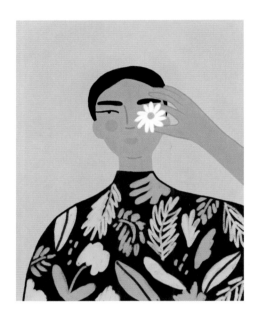

Sustainability

The beauty industry is one of the worst culprits for non-recyclable componentry and excess plastic packaging. It's important to keep raising the subject because that's how change happens; by people like you and me making lots of noise. According to Recycle Now, while 90% of Brits recycle kitchen waste, 50% don't recycle their bathroom packaging. As a result, they say, about 2.7 billion plastic bottles hit landfill every year in the UK alone.

Here are the worst beauty packaging offenders (in no particular order):

- Cellophane wrapping. The plastic straw of the beauty industry, this wrapping is totally unnecessary. Both the skincare and fragrance industries are guilty of "glossing" their boxes in cellophane to make them look more "prestige". This needs to stop, and it will only stop if we stop buying.

- Metal springs within shampoo and body lotion pumps. Unfortunately these springs are built into plastic pumps and can't be separated for recycling.

- Fold-out paperwork packed inside skincare boxes with detailed instructions and information in 200 different languages. The good news is that this waste of paper can now be avoided.

Brands such as Dior have started replacing them with scannable QR codes. Hurrah.

- Velvet and leather pouches. Once you've repurposed four of them to store kirby grips it's hard to think of uses for any more of them.

- Sealed packaging that can't be opened to wash out and recycle once you have got down to the last dregs of the product.

- Black plastic packaging inserts that can't be recycled because the optical scanners at recycling plants can't pick them out.

What can you do to aid the packaging crusade?

Andrew McDougall, Associate Director of Beauty & Personal Care at Mintel, points out: "Plastic is not inherently bad, but our throwaway use of it is." So the best practice might be, where possible, to avoid packaging altogether. If we make good decisions at the point of purchase, it will be easier for us to be kinder to the planet further down the line.

◇ We can buy soaps, cleansers and shampoos that come in bar form and can be picked up unwrapped (many shampoo bars are based on an animal fat, though, so watch out, vegans).

◇ Seek out glass jars that can be recycled indefinitely, or reused, or better still refilled (plenty of brands, from Aveda to MAC and Origins, will offer this service). That said, glass is not always the answer, since it is heavier and takes more energy to transport and therefore has a bigger carbon footprint than some plastic.

◇ Use recycling amnesty services. Garnier and Noble Panacea ensure your empties are recycled correctly.

◇ Look for brands that manufacture only with recycled or waste plastic, like RE=COMB.

◇ If you must buy plastic packaging, look for ocean-recycled plastic and avoid tiny componentry elements that jam up recycling machines.

◇ According to the EcoLife website, the safest way to get rid of old cosmetics is to carefully remove makeup from containers and put it all in a sealed jar or packaging that you can then send to landfill. That way, no harmful chemicals can leak out.

Also look out for the following symbols and terms:

Chasing arrows symbol: A triangle of arrows which contains a number that indicates how easy the product is to recycle, dependent on the type of plastic used to fabricate it. Products numbered 1–2 are easy, 3–5 are more complicated but doable, and 6–7 are difficult or impossible to reuse.

Sub-zero waste packaging: This is packaging that lives on for another purpose: for example, shampoo bottles that are embedded with seeds and can be planted in the garden.

Naked packaging: A fun buzzword for beauty products that are completely packaging-free, such as wax-coated foundation bars and shampoo bars.

Reef-friendly: This applies to packaging or ingredients that won't damage or clog up the ocean's reefs or disrupt its ecosystems.

Sustainability isn't all about packaging, however. Another big issue is carbon footprint. Once you've bought your essence from South Korea and ordered your konjac sponge from Japan, you've covered a fair few air miles. And it's not just shipping of final products: many brands use ingredients from far-flung origins, so your face cream has travelled extensive mileage before you've even bought it. As with food, it's important to think about shopping for your beauty products locally. British brands Bamford, Bee Good, Elemental Herbology, Neal's Yard and Noble Isle, for example, all source their ingredients from the UK.

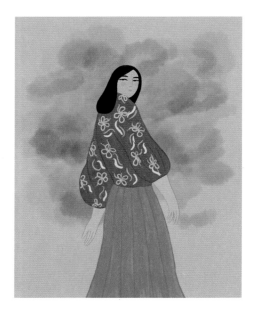

Anti-Pollution is
the New Anti-Ageing

The beauty industry loves to galvanize against a common enemy. We obsess over anything that's prefixed with the word "anti" (think anti-ageing, anti-stress, anti-blue light), and the latest cause is definitely "anti-pollution".

This comes as no surprise when you consider that, by 2050, 66% of the global population will live in cities, according to the United Nations. Air pollution is a massive threat (the Health Effects Institute has noted that air pollution is the fourth largest threat to human health after high blood pressure, dietary risks and smoking, and caused 4.2 million people around the world to die prematurely in 2015), but it is seriously bad news for our skin as well.

Why? Well, microscopic pollution particles from industry emissions – much smaller than your pores – can easily infiltrate the skin. Once inside, they trigger the formation of free-radical particles. These then break apart the cellular structure, causing inflammation and speeding up the ageing process. Toxic air is also linked to eczema, hives, and a special type of pollution-clogged acne that I call "urban acne".

The following are my anti-pollution skincare rules to live by:

◇ Protect your skin from pollution particles as you would from the sun.

◇ Cleanse your skin as soon as you step through the door in the evening, and then immediately apply your serum.

◇ Add a decongestant in the evening to deep-clean skin. I love This Works' Evening Detox Spray-on Exfoliant (which contains salicylic acid and witch hazel). As a decongesting mask I adore the Omorovicza Ultramoor Mud Mask (great for guys, too).

Anti-pollution products mostly tackle the fall-out from traffic and industrial emissions, but there are other environmental pollutants that dermatologists warn about. Blue light, or high-energy visible light (HEVL), is another big threat. Blue light is the glare that your smartphone and other digital screens emit, which has been proven to speed up the ageing process as well as stimulating an increase in pigmentation in skin. According to research by dermatologist-loved brand Skinceuticals, the hyperpigmentation triggered by HEVL is worse in black skin tones, which will see an increase of 18.3%, as opposed to 4.3% in light to medium skin tones. Then there's electromagnetic radiation (EMR), emitted from objects such as microwaves, which is also reported to age the skin.

Today's skincare offering is flooded with ingredients being labelled as "anti-pollution molecules" or "anti-pollution technology", but what does that really mean?

• It could be a reference to prebiotics or other ingredients that help culture the microbiome on the surface of the skin, which strengthens the defensive skin barrier.

• It could be an umbrella term for antioxidants, which are substances that help repair and defend skin cells from the free-radical damage generated by pollution particles.

• It could also be a reference to a "second skin", i.e. anti-pollution molecules that form a physical barrier over the skin. This is a hot topic, and such products are being pitched as the new sunscreens. Some brands describe them as a "mesh" or a "shield".

• In the future, anti-pollution products could be awarded a PPF – the SPF of pollution, essentially a potential, as yet unratified, system for quantifying pollution protection in skincare. A lower PPF value would refer to products that filter out a low percentage of pollution; a higher value would refer to higher levels of screening. Watch this space.

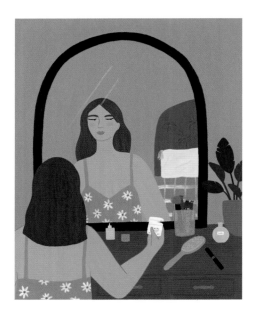

Dupes and Fakes

Fakery is commonplace in the beauty industry. Fake noses, fake freckles, fake followers... But there are two specific types of fake beauty that I want to talk about here: beauty dupes and counterfeit cosmetics.

A dupe refers to a knock-off of a prestige beauty product. You can find them everywhere: online, in drugstores or chemists, markets and supermarkets. Calling out these dupes has become a pastime of beauty bloggers, 'grammers and subreddit forums. There's even a vigilante-style Instagram account that names and shames shameless copycat brands: @esteelaundry. But dupes are mostly fairly harmless, and are sometimes actually quite brilliant. Aldi, for example, sells a line of home fragrances that are

strikingly similar to a certain black-and-cream-packaged British perfume brand at a couple of quid a pop; and who wouldn't be thrilled to get a nearly-but-not-quite designer skincare product for a tenth of the price?

But people are divided between whether dupes are ethically OK or not. Here are some of the arguments you might want to consider before purchasing a dupe.

An Argument for Skincare Dupes

- They democratize the beauty space, making products affordable for all. Shouldn't we all be able to access decent skincare? Don't the big beauty brands make enough money?

- Most skincare products are made in the same handful of factories, so the likelihood is that even the expensive brands are sharing ingredients and ideas at a top level anyway.

- It doesn't cost much to make a skincare cream, regardless of the ingredients, and brands tend to place a huge mark-up on their products. Dupes are often so cheap because they don't have such huge mark-ups.

- Dupes aren't illegal. Yes, they're lacking in imagination, but they are brought to market under the same formulation and safety requirements as any other product. They don't violate patent or copyright laws, so they shouldn't be considered in the same category as counterfeit or fake cosmetics (products that not only rip off the design but also the brand logo and other characteristics in order to trick consumers).

An Argument Against Skincare Dupes

- By buying a dupe, you are condoning the right for lazy brands to rip off other people's hard work and ingenuity.

- The more you spend on homogeneous copycat products, the less money you are putting into unique, independent brands that are encouraging creative talent.

- Less quality and care go into the ingredients selections for dupes. It's one thing in makeup, but in skincare quality of ingredient really does matter, and you will see a difference in your skin.

- It's a waste. There's enough plastic and chemicals in the world without making more.

- We can assume that good-quality, effective formulations require a considerable amount of research — an amount that would not be possible to recreate in the speed that most dupes are brought to market — and therefore it is likely that dupes on the whole are not brilliantly formulated.

Wherever you land on dupes, counterfeit skincare products are definitely a big problem in beauty. Faux no! Similar to fake fashion, they are bad for the beauty economy, they potentially employ workers who don't have access to rights and fair pay, they fund global crime, but on top of this — and what makes a fake lipstick potentially more dangerous than a fake handbag — is that they are often swarming with bacteria, cause allergic reactions, and even contain shards of glass.

Consider the following:

- Counterfeits may be formulated with ingredients that are not legal or not safety-approved by official regulations.

- They may be formulated in illegal labs alongside other ingredients that could be hazardous for the skin.

- They may be genuine products with safe ingredients, but are being re-sold illegally, and therefore they may have been stored in unsafe or unhygienic warehouses or in temperatures that make the ingredients go off.

- They may have been stored illegally for too long, pushing them past their sell-by date.

- At worst they might contain arsenic, rat poison, heavy metals, glass, and other toxic or skin-irritating substances. Nice.

Spotting a Fake

Thanks to the internet, beauty fakes are getting harder to spot, while being much easier to get hold of. Aside from sales on eBay and other marketplace sites, they are being shifted en masse on the dark web, an uncontrollable digital platform that allows the trade of counterfeit goods without the watchful eye of customs agents. That's right: on the dark web you can buy guns, drugs and lipstick!

My advice is always to shop your beauty from credible, reputable outlets – whether that's online or in-store. Contact a brand's customer service if you think you may have been sold counterfeit goods online, as many companies have entire departments dedicated to tracking fakes. Your sleuthing could actually help them out, while stopping other consumers just like you being fobbed off or endangered.

A raft of new cyber-security start-ups have also sprung up in response to the murky world of online cosmetic counterfeits. Entrupy is the world's first online authentication service to use "computer vision", which allows computers to capture microscopic surface data of packaging; they even have an app that allows brands to identify fakes of their products. Another start-up, DataWeave, can detect makeup counterfeits listed on e-commerce websites by identifying inconsistencies in the catalogue content and images, and by analysing sellers, prices and customer reviews.

Beauty Editor Tip
—

"Look for obvious typos in the brand name or slight discrepancies in the logo – 'MAP' instead of 'MAC', for example – or even something as tiny as a shade-name inaccuracy, such as 'Ruby Woah' instead of 'Ruby Woo'."

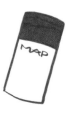

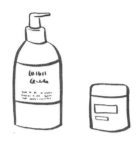

Beauty Editor Tip

—

"When you open the lid, does the product smell, look and feel right? Be especially wary of products that look as if they have curdled, or that smell much more synthetically fragranced than when you have bought them in the past."

Beauty Editor Tip

—

"If the product is insanely discounted (and by that I mean unbelievably cheap), this should be a red flag that the product may not be legit. Brands take counterfeits very seriously, so never worry about contacting them to check."

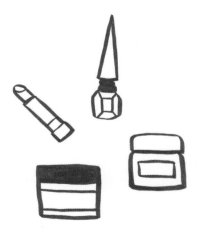

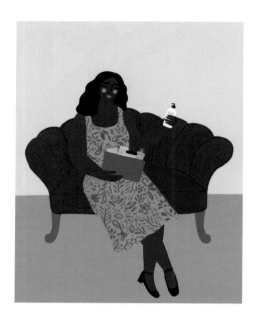

Use-By Dates and Preservatives

All beauty products expire. Just like foodstuffs, they have a use-by date. This is because, although most beauty products contain preservatives, those preservatives have a use-by date – and once they have stopped functioning, the product can start to break down and harbour bacteria and fungi. So that cleanser that's been lurking at the back of your bathroom cabinet? Yup, that probably needs to be thrown away.

"The lifecycle of a product is based on how long the preservatives can last. So if your product says it's suitable for use for twelve months but you're using it three years later, then the preservative system likely no longer works. 'Preservative-free' has become a marketing term that has led people to believe that a product having preservatives is a bad thing, which is troubling. On the other hand, I do like the fact that it challenges the industry to find different ways of preserving products."

Florence Adepoju, Cosmetic Scientist and Founder of MDMflow

Here are some commonly asked questions on how long your skincare can and should last:

How can I find out a product's use-by date?

You know that little icon on the back of your skincare that looks like a jar outline, with the lid opening, with a number inside it next to the letter M? Well, that number signifies the number of months you can keep using the product after opening it. So 6M would mean that you can keep using the product for six months before throwing it away. I know, mind-blowing. This icon is called a POA (period after opening). In the US, it's only a legal requirement for some products, but not all; in the UK, it's a legal requirement.

How stringently should I follow a use-by date?

How much do you want an eye infection? Seriously, you should be quite strict when it comes to following them.

Will a beauty fridge preserve my face cream for longer?

The demand for "fresh", less processed skincare is growing among natural beauty and wellbeing aficionados, and with it the trend for beauty fridges, i.e. mini fridges that you keep in your bathroom, as opposed to storing your serums and creams in the kitchen fridge. And while it may seem like a gimmick, generally keeping your products at a lower temperature *will* help preserve them. Cool temperatures will also slow down oxidation reactions, which are common in makeup especially. You shouldn't keep your natural oils in a fridge, though, as it messes with their consistency.

What natural preservatives are there out there?

There are quite a few natural preservatives that are used in cosmetics, but unfortunately none of them will preserve the shelf life of a product for long in comparison with synthetic preservatives. Some examples are lemon, salt, rosemary, potassium sorbate, vitamin E and citric acid. You can also get organic acids as preservatives, which are considered natural but are actually made synthetically.

What products tend to have the shortest shelf life?

Products that have a high water content tend to have a shorter shelf life, since water encourages the growth of bacteria. Powder-based products will last longest because they have no or minimal water content.

Are natural preservatives as efficient as synthetic ones?

Unfortunately they are not. Synthetic preservatives such as parabens (see also p. 37) and phenoxy-ethanol can hold a product stable for a considerably longer time, hence they are the safer (and much cheaper) option for most non-natural brands.

Do synthetic preservatives cause cancer?

This is a really difficult question. There are concerns over carcinogenic activity when it comes to some (though not all) synthetic preservatives, especially parabens and phenoxyethanol. The study on parabens was disputed, but the bad press has been enough to put people off products that contain them, and many brands now market themselves as "paraben-free" or "synthetic-preservative-free".

How can I tell if a product has gone off?

The smell, the appearance and the texture may have changed. Or you may experience a breakout or a rash when you apply the product due to a build-up of bacteria.

What are the main concerns with using a skincare product that has gone out of date?

Aside from the risk of breakouts, fungal infections and skin irritations, you need to be careful because active ingredients such as SPFs could cease functioning, meaning your skin is more vulnerable to major damage. "When in doubt, leave it out", as we say in the magazine world.

1

Get the Glossary

The Essentials of Good Skincare

As a beauty editor, I see anything between five and fifteen new skincare products a week. That's a staggering amount of lotions and potions filling up the shelves every year. Just when you think you've grasped the latest super-ingredient or masking technique, something else has launched, claiming to be better. But while beauty fads may come and go, certain terms appear again and again. So here, to help you comprehend the complexities of "beauty speak" – both scientific terminology and marketing spiel – is my beauty editor cheat sheet. Get to grips with these words and phrases and you'll sound convincingly in the know and hopefully stand a better chance of buying something that will actually work for your skin.

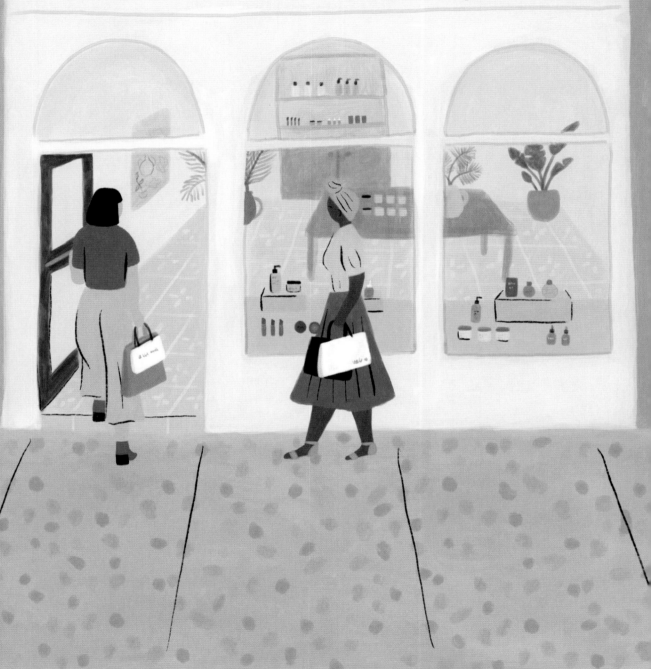

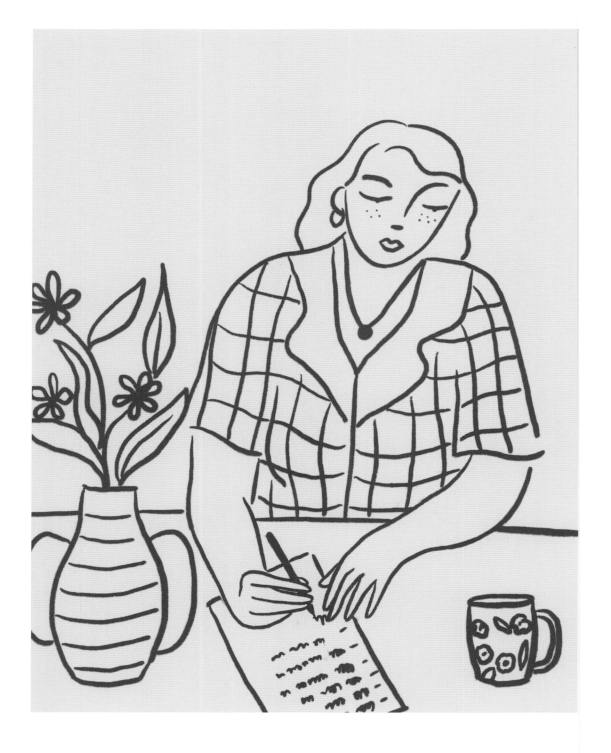

Ingredients to Know

Algae

This slimy sea organism caught the attention of cosmetic scientists a while back due to its impressive environmental resilience. Algae survives, even flourishes, in some of the darkest, coldest, most inhospitable environments in the world. There's a lot we can learn from it when it comes to making our skin more resilient. There are over 200,000 different species but, in general, when algae is used in **anti-ageing** skincare (see p. 53) it's for its protective moisturization, anti-inflammatory and **antioxidant** (see below) properties. Varieties to look out for are blue-green algae (spirulina), vitamin-rich chlorella, and intertidal seaweed algae which contains a rare amino acid that triggers skin's **collagen** repair process (see p. 30) and strengthens the skin barrier.

Antioxidants

Much referenced in skincare adverts, these are rarely explained. They are substances (often vitamins) that inhibit a breakdown process in our bodies called oxidation by free radicals, which causes our skin to age. The best demo I was ever shown was of a face serum containing antioxidants being applied to one of two slices of apple that were then left out on a plate. The slice without the antioxidant serum went brown within minutes, and the slice with the serum on remained fresh and juicy. The antioxidants had neutralized the free radicals that caused the apple to turn brown.

Bamboo Extract

Traditionally used in Chinese medicine for skin healing, bamboo is a source of **antioxidants** (above) but not a particularly strong one. I prefer to recommend bamboo grains as a great, eco alternative to plastic microbeads in physical face scrubs. Its Latin name, so you can spot it on the **INCI list** (see p. 168), is *Bambusa vulgaris*.

Blue Zone

Blue Zone ingredients are botanicals that promote skin longevity, found in five locations around the world known for their high concentration of centenarians: Okinawa (Japan), Ikaria (Greece), Ogliastra (Sardinia), Loma Linda (California) and the Nicoya Peninsula (Costa Rica). Chanel and Bare Minerals both have great products with ingredients from Blue Zones. Ingredients include the Long Life Herb from Japan, olives from Sardinia, and green coffee from Costa Rica.

Caffeine

You'd be forgiven for assuming that caffeine had the same reviving function in face cream as an espresso shot, but interestingly caffeine has been found to be fantastic at reducing **inflammation** (see p. 127), and is consequently a great treatment for dermatitis and psoriasis – two of the most chronic skin conditions.

Caviar

The fish egg itself isn't used in skincare but rather extracts from the omega- and amino acid-rich matrix that surrounds it (La Prairie have found a way of doing this without killing the fish). Does it work? The hefty price tag would suggest it does, but there isn't much conclusive research behind it. Then again, sometimes the placebo of luxury is all you need.

CBD (Cannabidiol)

The part of the cannabis plant that contains no THC (the hallucinogen) is completely legal in most countries and has been proven in clinical studies to have an anti-inflammatory response in the skin. We actually have cannabinoid receptors naturally in our body. You'll see CBD cropping up in face creams all over the shop...

Ceramides

Ceramides are unsung heroes, first and foremost because they are universally great rejuvenators for all skin types. These little-shouted-about lipids (good fats) make up over 50% of our skin's composition at birth, a number that depletes as we age from as early as our twenties. Ceramides surround our skin cells, like mortar to bricks, helping to retain moisture within the structure of the skin and keeping its texture all plump and marshmallowy. Elizabeth Arden's ceramide capsules are a favourite of mine because they are so easy to travel with and extremely reliable for instantly comfy skin.

Cica

Dry cracked hands, meet your saviour. Cica repair creams, balms and **lotions** (see p. 41) are formulated with a traditional Chinese botanical called *Centella asiatica* or tiger grass, so-called because tigers in the wild roll around in the stuff when they have wounds to heal. There are lots of wonderful Eastern mythologies about princes and warriors discovering tiger grass, but essentially all you need to know is that it is second to none for restoring cracked, irritated skin. The best ones are from French pharmacy brands like Mixa and La Roche Posay.

"I am a firm believer in Ayurvedic principles, which prescribe to the benefits of *Centella asiatica* as an antioxidant. I have found this to be a fail-safe go-to ingredient - particularly via moisturizers - for my fair (i.e. thin), sensitive skin."

Mia Collins, Head of Beauty, Harrods

Coffee Beans

Coffee is a natural **antioxidant** (see p. 29), but it's the discarded post-cappuccino grounds that are really causing a stir in beauty circles. The UK alone sends 500,000 tonnes of coffee to landfill each year, but one clever bodycare brand, Optiat, has begun collecting grounds from baristas all over London to repurpose into natural body scrubs. Genius.

Collagen

A protein found in the connective tissues all over the body, collagen is stronger than steel by weight; it quite literally holds us together. From our mid-twenties, supplies of it start to deplete by about 1% each year. Hello, skin sagging and wrinkles. Unfortunately, collagen creams aren't the most effective answer, and nor are collagen drinks. Look instead for ingredients that kick-start collagen production in the skin such as copper, **retinol** (see p. 112) and **vitamin C** (see p. 39), as these are a much more efficient, proven solution (and a better option for vegans, since collagen is sourced from animals and there are no plant-based sources).

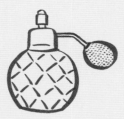

Fragrance

Beauty brands aren't legally obliged to disclose their scent molecules and often don't, simply listing "fragrance" or "parfum". Generally speaking, fragrance in skincare has two purposes: for sensory effect to please the user (have you ever tested a face cream on the back of your hand and not smelled it?) or to mask the farmyard smell of the actual ingredients. Fragrances can be natural (often from **essential oils**; see p. 83) or synthetic (made in a lab). Most creams, even natural ones, have them added separately. Neither natural nor synthetic come problem-free, as both can be potentially irritating to sensitive skin. That's why "fragrance-free" products are often recommended by dermatologists (according to the American Academy of Dermatology, fragrance is the biggest cause of cosmetic contact dermatitis). If you don't see the words "fragrance" or "parfum" on the label, have a look for linalool or citronellol, which are other commonly added scents.

"Any cream with a very strong smell is most likely synthetic. Natural materials on the skin generally smell very soft. All raw materials smell, though, so if your product is unscented what most people won't realize is that it contains a fragrance inhibitor as an additive."

Roja Dove, Perfumer

Geranium

In aromatherapy, this earthy-smelling **essential oil** (see p. 83) is celebrated for its stress-relieving and anti-depressive properties.

"It's easy to love geranium. First and foremost, it has a beautiful smell. You only have to rub the leaves of the scented *Pelargonium graveolens* to feel a boost. It's uplifting and a tonic, but it's less known for its many therapeutic values. Dr Jean Valnet [one of the world's foremost authorities on essential oil therapy] writes that the Ancients regarded it as having

the power to mend fractures and eliminate cancers. No one today could make such claims. Valnet's less controversial recipes include infusions to soothe chicken pox, herpes and eczema. Geranium is acknowledged to have anti-viral, anti-infectious and anti-spasmodic properties. Mostly, though, it's found as a balancing middle note in fine fragrances, bath oils and body lotions to give energy and to strengthen the resolve. A truly positive essential oil."

Kathy Phillips, ex-British *Vogue* Beauty Director, Author and Aromatherapy Expert

Ginger

You might see this listed under its Latin botanical name, *Zingiber officinale*. A bold statement, but if I had to pick one desert island botanical ingredient it would be ginger. It contains over forty **antioxidants** (see p. 29), and is anti-inflammatory and **anti-ageing** (see p. 53). In traditional Chinese medicine, ginger fills you with body-warming Yang energy, and it has been used for centuries to settle digestion, fight fatigue and boost motivation. It's one of the star ingredients in Dr Frances Prenna Jones's Formula, which is a brilliant everyday tonic for pepping up skin.

Beauty Editor Tip
—

"I like to fill gloomy Monday mornings with ginger. Two or three drops of essential oil in the bath, followed by a ginger-infused facial toner, a lemon and ginger tea, then a roll of ginger essential oil over the pulse points and under the nose as I step out the door for my commute. If essential oils were emojis, ginger would be the double high five."

Gold

"It's my opinion that gold, as an active ingredient, doesn't deliver on its promises as an anti-ageing, antioxidant or anti-inflammatory mineral for the skin. The amount actually used in formulations is so minimal, due to the cost of the raw ingredient, you aren't going to see results from it. You would need to smother your skin in gold to see any actual real results. I know Cleopatra would probably disagree with me, but I feel it's more of a gimmick than anything else. That said, as a reflective shimmer, nothing can beat it. Gold bounces light in just the right places to leave even the dullest and palest skin glowing, and who doesn't want that? In my opinion, if gold is one of the ingredients listed along with other more skin-benefitting ingredients, then it's doing no harm. If you're buying a product purely based on it containing gold, then I'd think about what you actually want from the product to ensure you aren't disappointed."

Haley Bloom Fitzpatrick, New Product Developer

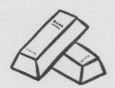

1. Get the Glossary

Glycerin, or Glycerol

A regular spot on ingredient labels, this is a **humectant** (see p. 51), which means it holds in water and gives many creams and **gels** (see p. 41) a smoother texture. Absolutely safe and harmless.

Grapes

Bursting with the super-antioxidant **resveratrol** (see p. 37), grapes also produce grape seed oil (usually from seeds discarded in the wine-making process), which contains twice as much **vitamin E** (see p. 39) as **olive oil** (see p. 91). In addition, it's high in linoleic acid, which is a brilliant **pore-minimizing** ingredient (see p. 62). Grape seeds can also be used in **scrubs** (see p. 43) as eco-exfoliants instead of plastic.

Hyaluronic Acid

This wonder moisturizer, which has hit peak popularity in recent years, is a water magnet. One hyaluronic acid molecule can hold up to 1,000 times its own weight in H2O. The beauty aisles are now abundant with HA serums, creams, **fake tans** (see p. 103), **sheet masks** (see p. 76) and concentrates, all of which are available in low, medium and high density, which essentially corresponds to the varying depths it can be helped to penetrate your skin.

"Hyaluronic acid is the unwavering ingredient on my hit list. I immediately notice a difference in my skin (both texture and volume) if I stop using it. I still remember the first time I tried a hyaluronic serum (the Dr Barbara Sturm ampoules). It was a 7-day course the week before my wedding and I was genuinely stunned by the results."

Mia Collins, Head of Beauty, Harrods

Beauty Editor Tip
—

"I like to keep an HA serum in my bag (La Roche Posay make a great one) to apply to my forehead, backs of hands and lips when they feel dry throughout the day. I also recommend hyaluronic foot creams to use in between pedicures."

Icelandic Water

Not all waters are created equal. Icelandic water is some of the "emptiest" water in the world because when rain falls on the land it trickles through the island's volcanic rock landscape, which acts as a natural filtration system.

"The water in Iceland is pumped from underground, and it is absolutely clean, natural and pure. There are no traces of agrochemicals, nor of heavy metals which are bad for the skin as they can catalyse free-radical production. The water also contains little to no calcium, so it is very soft and therefore gentler on the skin and easier to cleanse with, requiring less soap."

Dr Björn Örvar, PhD in Plant-Molecular Biology and Co-founder of Bioeffect

Kale

Everyone's favourite superfood is a vitamin powerhouse. Vitamin K is used topically in creams that claim to treat rosacea, stretch marks, spider veins and post-procedure scarring. The jury's out, though, as to whether applying it in a cream will actually do any good, and more research is needed. For now, experts place better bets on sticking it in your salad. One cup of cooked kale offers 53.3 mg of **collagen**-stimulating **vitamin C** (see pp. 30 and 39), which is nothing to be scoffed at.

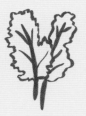

Liposomes

These spherical sacs are used to transport cosmetic ingredients or nutrients deep into the skin, like tiny Deliveroo drivers ferrying tiny burgers to starving skin cells. They manage to penetrate the skin so efficiently because skin cells recognize their shape as identical to the lipids already existing in the skin. Very clever.

Magnesium

A very useful mineral indeed, magnesium is responsible for hundreds of natural processes in the body functioning correctly, including circulation, muscle repair, and even DNA synthesis. Not surprisingly then there are a lot of magnesium-based beauty products on the market, from bath flakes to oils and sprays, and even anti-acne creams. Many of these are in my opinion brilliant (I love a post-yoga magnesium bath), but be warned they can tend to oversell their effectiveness. According to some studies, there is doubt over how easily magnesium can penetrate the skin. It's been proven that it definitely permeates through the hair follicle and sweat glands, but not in vast quantities. Popping a pill may be more effective.

Manuka Honey

This antibacterial, healing honey is produced in New Zealand by bees that pollinate the manuka bush. Not all manuka honey is sustainably sourced, and not all of it is the high quality its price tag promises it to be. Look for brands that use manuka honey with an MGO rating of 300+ to be sure you're getting the good stuff.

"Manuka honey is one of Mother Nature's wonder ingredients. It contains an occurring enzyme that produces hydrogen peroxide which is natural. This is a known antiseptic with antibacterial and antimicrobial properties. From these findings, manuka honey is used for wound care in hospitals. It can help stimulate the immune system, provide nutrients for cell metabolism, reduce inflammation, and aid rapid tissue repair."

Haley Bloom Fitzpatrick, New Product Developer

Matcha

A souped-up version of **green tea** (see p. 74), matcha contains high levels of an **antioxidant** (see p. 29) called epigallocatechin gallate (which someone has kindly abbreviated to EGCG). There is little concrete evidence that matcha is better for your skin when applied via a cream than simply green tea extract, so don't get stung with a hefty price tag just because it's trendy.

Manuka Honey

"Manuka honey is amazing. Sometimes I use
it to make a mask if my skin is really
tired or if I'm really stressed. Stress
will make your skin defensive, as in
harder and dryer. So manuka honey will
work to soften that skin on the surface.
Sometimes I just slap it straight on! It's
a bit sticky, and it can be a bit messy,
but it's such a nice thing to do and you
can almost feel it loving your skin. It's
like a big hug from a bee!"

Nichola Joss, Facialist

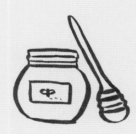

Parabens

"Parabens are super-cheap. They are also super-easy to formulate with, since you only need the tiniest amount. As a result, they don't impact the formula as much as other preservatives do.

They also don't have a strong colour base, which is why I find they are good for formulating for women of colour, as they won't impact the colour of your skin."

Florence Adepoju, Cosmetic Scientist and Founder of MDMflow

Niacinamide

Otherwise known as vitamin B3, and also referred to as nicotinic acid (but nothing to do with nicotine), this is the go-to ingredient if you're trying to reduce the appearance of enlarged pores. It also works wonders on smoothing out hyperpigmentation, thus being an excellent choice for darker skin tones that are prone to pigmentation or scarring.

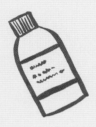

Parabens

A type of preservative, parabens have a terrifically bad rep thanks mostly to a 2004 British study, which found traces of them in the breast tissue of 19 out of 20 women being screened for breast cancer. The study isn't proof that parabens cause cancer, but it was enough to spook most discerning beauty enthusiasts. Despite the bad press, parabens are still found in 75% of all cosmetics globally (in everything from shower gels to shampoos and moisturizers) and remain Food and Drug Administration-approved, so companies that scaremonger them as "toxic" are being opinionated as opposed to strictly factual. Where there is smoke, though, there may be fire, so if you can avoid them, I would. Look out for the commonly used butylparaben, methylparaben and propylparaben the back of the label.

Propolis

This bee by-product is made from tree sap and used by bees in the hive to keep out fungi and bad bacteria. It's a really nice natural alternative to many of the quite harsh **acne** (see p. 127) treatments on the market, since propolis is both antibacterial and antifungal.

Quinoa Husks

Off-cuts from quinoa production in South and Central America, these husks make amazing chemical exfoliators, so you'll find them used in overnight **essences** (see p. 74) and at-home skin peels. Kiehl's does a great one.

Resveratrol

Arguably the best **antioxidant** (see p. 29) on the market, resveratrol is a polyphenol (a protective substance produced by plants when they come under stress). Studies have found that 1% resveratrol applied topically yielded a "statistically significant improvement" in wrinkles, radiance, hyperpigmentation, skin roughness, firmness and elasticity in just over twelve weeks. There is also strong evidence that it works wonders on **acne** (see p. 127), and convincing studies show that it is a skin cancer anticarcinogen. You'll find it in **grape** extract (see p. 33).

Beauty Editor Tip
—
"You can also find resveratrol in supplement form at health retailers. Supplements are clinically proven to reduce the depth of your wrinkles."

Rose

As an essential oil, rose is used in skincare for its calming and soothing properties. The holy trinity in gold-standard rose skincare consists of Damascan rose, Rose de Mai and Moroccan rose. These may knock the price bracket of your purchase up but will allow you to reap the best rewards. Other rose variants to look out for are rosehip seed oil, which comes from the small fruit behind the rose flower and is packed with **vitamins A** (see p. 112), D, **C** and **E** (see p. 39), and rosewater, which is created from a distillation of rose oil in water and makes a great addition to a cleansing or **micellar** water (see p. 41).

Beauty Editor Tip
—
"My pick of the crop when it comes to rose products is the Ila Day Cream for Glowing Radiance. I use it religiously during the winter months."

Silicones

A good guy often painted as a bad guy, silicones are used in creams, serums, foundations, primers and shampoos to manufacture that incredible, sliding, silky smooth feeling. There are over 2,000 different forms, and though they are man-made they are actually naturally derived from silica (sand).

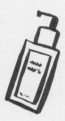

"There's so much science behind silicone technology, and there are so many different types of silicones and so many different usages. Can they clog pores? That depends on the quality of the silicone, how it's been synthesized and the particle size, because if you put anything of a large particle size on top of pores it's going to block them to a certain extent, even if it's a natural-based ingredient. Personally, I love formulating lipsticks with silicone-treated pigments in my lipstick brand."

Florence Adepoju, Cosmetic Scientist and Founder of MDMflow

1. Get the Glossary

Sodium Lauryl Sulphate

This is a foaming agent, meaning its main purpose is to generate satisfying bubbles. It is openly classified as an irritant, and can be extremely drying on skin. Worryingly, SLS is still used in a vast array of shampoos, washes and cleansers, despite a survey by health food store Holland & Barrett that found 41% of women were unaware of SLS's existence in cosmetics at all.

Turmeric

Do not, whatever you do, apply neat turmeric to your skin directly. No matter what you see on Instagram, or what you read about turmeric's bona fide anti-inflammatory properties, it will stain your skin a garish shade of yellow. Take a supplement instead. Turmeric is a fantastic anti-inflammatory, so it's great for minimizing **acne** swelling (see p. 127) and other skin irritations.

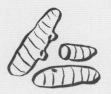

Vitamin C

Berocca for the complexion? Vitamin C is commonly found in **anti-pollution** skin creams (see pp. 18 and 97) and products whose purpose is to even, brighten and smooth skin tone. It's also used to help treat photodamaged skin (aka skin that has been exposed to too much sun).

Vitamin E

Another **antioxidant** (see p. 29), this is a great moisturizer/skin healer and is often recommended for scarring. On the label you'll see it written as d-alpha-tocopherol, d-alpha-tocopherol acetate, dl-alpha tocopherol or dl-alpha tocopherol acetate. The letter "d" as a prefix indicates it was derived from natural sources, "dl" from synthetic; it's thought that natural forms are more effective than synthetic. See also p. 121.

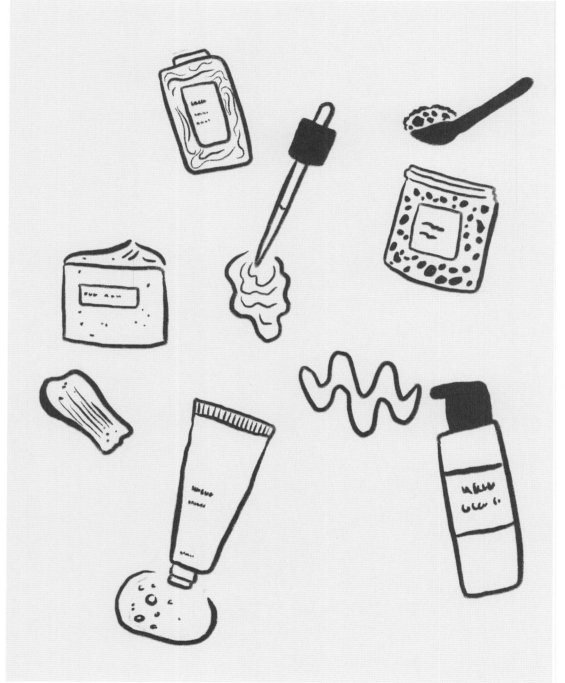

Textures

Crème

Aka cream. Nothing fancy, just "cream" said in a French accent by skincare brands who want to make their tub of moisturizer sound a bit posher and worth the hefty price tag they're flogging it for. Always makes me laugh.

Emulsion

Scientifically speaking, an emulsion is a stable blend of an oil and water. In skincare it's often used to describe something that's lighter than a thick moisturizing cream but a bit thinner than a **lotion** (see right).

Gel

Most gels are formulated to please: they feel lighter, fresher, more thirst-quenching and less greasy than oil-based creams. Marketing teams decided long ago, rather patronisingly, that gels suited men's ranges, which is why you'll find most male-gendered skincare lines centre around man-gels. I like to keep mine in the fridge or pop them in the freezer five minutes before use (just don't forget they're in there!). Gels are brilliant for oily skin types, and in fact most skincare ranges worth their salt will include a gel version of their hero moisturizer. Look for gels that list **dimethicone** (a type of **silicone**; see pp. 61 and 38) in the first few ingredients, as this will prevent water from evaporating from the skin, keeping it hydrated for longer.

Intensive Cream, or Crème Intensive

This is used to describe hi-tech creams that contain substantial concentrations of **active** ingredients (see p. 49). A little red flag should pop up here, though. The word "intensive", or its French translation "intensif" (see **crème** above), is often just marketing. Always check the back of the label for more clues on how concentrated the formula really is.

Lotion

Positioned alongside **crèmes** and **soufflés** (see above and p. 43), lotions can feel a bit "basic", conjuring up depressing images of changing rooms at the gym. On the other hand, they go a little bit further than thicker body creams or **gels** (see left), making them more economic, plus – for the same reason, i.e. they are more aqueous – they leave skin less sticky.

Beauty Editor Tip
—
"In the hot weather, when thicker creams become more of a burden, I switch to using a liposome lotion (I love the one by Decorté). All the refreshing feels of a lightweight lotion with the brilliant technology of liposome nutrient delivery systems."

Micellar Water

This makeup-removing liquid consists of "micelles", or tiny spheres of cleansing oil suspended in water. It's just so practical, and allows you to be extremely lazy with your skincare regime while actually doing quite a good job of keeping skin clean and hydrated.

"I always finish off my skincare regime with a floral mist. It was a tip from my friend, makeup artist Tom Pecheux. And I use a rose water mist to wake up the skin every day before going out."

Montasar Dumas, Communication Manager, Shiseido and Clé de Peau Beauté

Milk

Similar to **lotions** (see p. 41), milks are thin-textured moisturizers. They do not, and should not, contain actual milk (although some people do rave about bathing in cows' milk). If you enjoy using bath oils, then I recommend trying an aromatherapeutic-grade bath milk. Regular bath oils float on the surface of the bath water, meaning that although you inhale the aromatherapy benefits, they are unlikely to affect the skin submerged under the water. Bath milks, on the other hand, are **emulsions** (see p. 41) that can diffuse through the water, meaning that the **essential oils** (see p. 83) will permeate the whole bath tub and can be far more effectively therapeutic for problems like achy muscles and dry skin. Value for money approved.

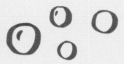

Mousse

These aerated liquids are either dispensed through an aerosol (bad for the environment) or through a pump (better for the environment, so long as you take it apart when it's empty and recycle the bits that you can). Some brands make mousse primers or foundations, but the bubbles have no effect on efficacy.

Mud

Mud, glorious mud! I wonder who first discovered that rolling around in mud had skincare benefits? Certain muds (let's be clear that not all muds are beautifying) contain buckets of trace minerals that work together to minimize the appearance of pores, calm **inflammation** (see p. 127), even out skin tone, and exfoliate and **detoxify** (see p. 53) oily skin. Quite often the word "mud" will be used on the front of the packet but the mask will actually list a **clay** (see p. 133).

Mist

This is a skincare **lotion** (see p. 41), water or **essence** (see p. 74) that is vaporized or spritzed on application. In my opinion, several things are infinitely superior when used in mist form. **Fake tan** (see p. 103) mists, for example, are a genius invention; suncream, too. It halves application time and keeps your hands mess-free. You can even get mist-on **toners** (see p. 104) and moisturizers, which are excellent for on-the-go beauty.

Scrub

Scrubs have inadvertently become one of beauty's most contentious products. The humble exfoliator came under vast scrutiny for commonly containing microbeads, the now banned plastic spheres that were escaping down the drain and into the ocean. But happily there are plenty of kinder-to-the-planet scrubbing agents on the market. To name just a few of my favourites: micronized **bamboo** (see p. 29), sugar, salt, **quinoa husks** (see p. 37), oats, kiwi seeds, and used **coffee** granules (see p. 30).

Soufflé

This whipped cream texture is employed purely for the novelty and pleasure of how it feels when it's applied. The link between beauty and dessert will pop up several times over the course of this book, especially when we come to Korean skincare (see p. 71).

"We all want skincare that works, and beauty brands are responsible for some of the most cutting-edge scientific research. My stash is full of serums backed up by science - I always recommend friends read up on the research before they buy. Stem cells, the dermis and collagen are our skin's health powerhouses, and they need to be looked after. I always pat in my serum, using the kind of pressure you'd use to test if a peach were ripe. The action of pressing into the skin rather than rubbing across makes the surface microscopically open, allowing the serum to absorb quicker and the goodness to get to work."

Olivia de Courcy, Beauty Editor

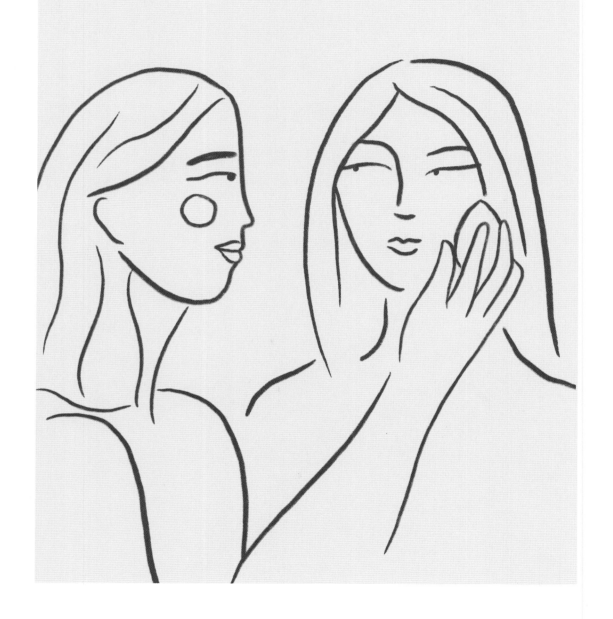

Techniques

Acid Toning

Everyday toning is all about balancing and restoring the skin's surface. Acid toning, however, combines a regular toner with an acid (less scary than it sounds) to exfoliate and hydrate at the same time as pH balancing. The advantages are fresher, clearer, more even-looking skin, removal of excess oil, and a real glow the following morning. For travel and ease many brilliant derm brands such as Zelens, Kate Somerville and Dr Colbert do handy pre-soaked acid toner pads. If you have sensitive skin, look for an acid toner that contains **PHA** (see p. 108) – a much gentler, more **hydrating** (see p. 54) variant.

Blending

The iconic Beauty Blender egg-shaped sponge is much copied, but the original has a pointed end to help apply skincare or makeup into the corners around the nose and eyes and a bigger, rounder end for the flatter planes of your face. Always wet the sponge first.

Double Cleansing

A practice that hails from Southeast Asia and South Korea, double cleansing uses two different cleansers one after the other. Worth it, or just another reason to spend more money? The theory behind double cleansing is that the first cleanse removes your makeup and any surface-level dirt using an oil-based cleanser, while the second cleanse with a **water-based** (see p. 57) or cream cleanser can more effectively clean the skin now the makeup has been lifted off. In my opinion, it's definitely worthwhile if you wear foundation or **SPF** (see p. 94) every day.

Eye Cream Application

You either love eye cream and apply it religiously or you just don't see the point. I fall into the latter camp, but God forbid I should stop you from spending your hard-earned cash on a tiny pot of cream that's basically just another moisturizer re-marketed... That said, the skin around the eyes is much thinner than the skin over the rest of the face and does need to be cared for with regular hydration and **detoxifying** (see p. 53) ingredients to look its best. Key ingredients to look for are: **vitamin C** (brightening; see p. 39) **aloe vera** (for reducing puffiness; see p. 123), **hyaluronic acid** (hydrating; see p. 33) and argireline (tightening). I've often been told by facialists not to apply heavy **eye cream at night** (see p. 103), as it may collect in the skin under your eyes overnight without being drained away, leaving you with puffy eyes in the morning.

Gankin Massage

Gankin is a Japanese facial pick-me-up massage technique, helping to firm, **detox** (see p. 53) and contour the face, all without the need for electric currents or massage devices.

"With just the pressure of your hands and a cream, massaging certain pressure points with a Gankin massage will awaken your face and quite literally give you cheekbones. I use it as a skin/face prep on actors at 5am before their makeup. We don't realize how much tension we carry in our faces, and it's a wonderful way to de-stress. Go as deep with the pressure as you can for best results."

Morag Ross, Movie Makeup Artist

Double Cleansing

"For the first cleanse I like to use a facial wash as opposed to an oil, and a lot of people would say that's just mad but I like to feel clean. The first cleanse will just remove most of the SPF and the foundation, and the second one I'll remove with a cotton pad just to ensure that all residue comes off. You're left with really, really clean skin, ready for treatment."

Teresa Tarmey, Facialist

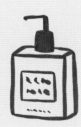

Inner Mouth Massage

This technique was developed by A-list facialist Nichola Joss, who dons her plastic gloves and massages your face from the inside of your mouth. It's reported to be a little painful but amazingly lifting. Fans of her inner mouth facial have included Angelina Jolie and Meghan Markle, to name a few.

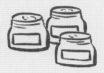

Multi-masking

Part Insta-trend, part genius skincare idea, multi-masking is the use of multiple different face masks over multiple parts of the skin at one time. The patchwork effect is infinitely Instagrammable — at the time of typing there are over 50,000 posts hashtagged under "multimasking" to prove it, each one as bizarre-looking as the next. This phenomenon is a skincare brand's ultimate dream — an opportunity to sell you four different types of face mask when previously one would do. When will we learn!? That said, multi-masking has caught on because it's actually quite clever. Different zones of our complexion behave differently and therefore require different treatment. My ultimate multi-mask regime is **kaolin clay** (see p. 76) over my nose to deep-clean my pores, **vitamin E** (see p. 39) over my chin where I have a scar that often peels, **hyaluronic acid** (see p. 33) over my forehead to quench my dehydration line, and a brightening anti-redness mask over my cheeks.

Steaming

Exposing your face to warm steam once a week (too hot or too often can be skin-irritating) in advance of cleansing will help loosen the sebum within the pores, making it easier to deep-clean. If you can't be bothered to stand over a sink with a hot flannel held up to your visage, why not just utilize the steam that comes off your morning shower.

"Sometimes I use steam to dilate the pores before extraction. The heat will make the pores dilate, but as soon as you take that steam away the cold will shrink the pores back again, so you have quite a short window. I'm not a massive fan of subjecting the skin to too much heat just to then start messing with it, though (I think it can cause aggravation), so you need to use steam with caution. A lactic acid peel to soften and remove dead skin is often a better alternative."

Teresa Tarmey, Facialist

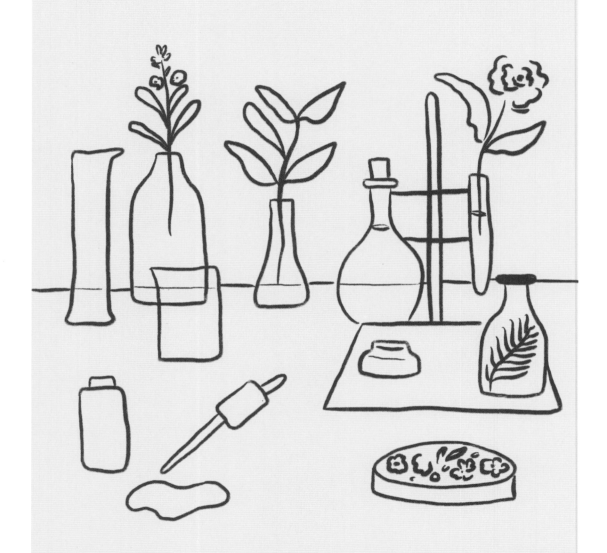

The Science

Active

The rock stars of the skincare world, active ingredients will actively make changes in the skin to fight free radicals, counter **inflammation** (see p. 127), and soothe, repair or stimulate various processes to make you look younger. Everything else in a formula is inactive, i.e. designed to deliver the actives into the skin, preserve the shelf life of the product, or give it a certain look, feel or smell.

Bio-identical

Scientists can clone natural ingredients in the lab and structurally, under a microscope, you couldn't tell the difference – they are identical – but in reality they will make quite a big difference to your skin. Bio-identicals have a much lower risk of allergy or causing skin irritation. Seeing "bio-identical" on the skincare label is a really good sign for the planet, too, as the ingredients are created without pillaging the world's natural resources. No rainforests are cut down to create space to grow them, no natural ecosystems are disturbed, and no pesticides are used. The greener ingredient choice for sure.

Bio-mimetic

These man-made beauty ingredients imitate natural ingredients in order to be accepted within the skin's structures. Consider the gatekeeper cells guarding the entrance to the lower levels of the skin as bouncers to a club, who will only let ingredients enter that have complied to a certain dress code.

Bio-fermented

So you're already a fan of kombucha and kimchi at lunchtime, but what can fermented ingredients do for your complexion? Well, the good news is that fermenting a natural ingredient can supercharge its potency and produce more **antioxidants** (see p. 29), giving you even better results. Fermenting is also a wonderfully sustainable way of "farming" skincare ingredients, as bio-ferments are produced in the lab and take less toll on the planet. Examples of ingredients that can be fermented are **hyaluronic acid** (see p. 33), sea kelp, **ginseng** (see p. 74) and soy.

Epigenetics

Relatively hard to explain in brief, but here goes... Our lifestyles and our experiences can over time cause our genes to switch on and off. The food you eat, the stress you put yourself under, the place you live, the type of exercise you do, it all can affect the way our genes behave and ultimately the way we age. Some pioneering skincare brands are now designing products with this in mind, either developing bespoke products that adapt to your unique gene map or products that seek to counter the negative effects that polluted environments and high-stress lifestyles have on our genes. At consumer level, epigenetic skincare is still in its infancy (so either not that advanced or astronomically expensive), but generally it's a very exciting concept.

Supplements

"I rely heavily on products and supplements to keep me looking like a semi-functional human woman. Since I started using Dr Dennis Gross Alpha Beta cleanser I don't really get spots, and I'm now horribly addicted to the appallingly expensive but peerless Augustinus Bader Rich Cream - on the upside I no longer use much concealer, on the downside I shall soon be bankrupt. My imminent insolvency has been compounded by the realization that what we ingest is the key to a reasonable complexion, so I rattle with top-quality vitamin D, omega oils, Bergatone, DIMs, Viviscal, nootropics and magnesium."

Annabel Rivkin, Journalist

Humectant

This moisturizing ingredient or compound found throughout skincare actively attracts moisture to it. Examples would be propylene glycol or **aloe vera gel** (see p. 123).

Micro-encapsulated

There are some ingredients that just don't like being absorbed into the lower levels of the skin, so formulators have discovered that these can be contained (micro-encapsulated) in tiny bubbles that act as taxi cabs for the ingredients, picking them up at the surface of your skin and dropping them off deep in the dermis so that they can be put to work where they're needed. Clever, huh? Another form of micro-encapsulation is where the bubbles contain **fragrance** (see p. 30) and are designed to burst while you're using the product so that the fragrance is released into the air.

Stem Cells

In the quest for eternal youth, stem cells are providing some exciting answers. The role of stem cells within the skin is to produce specialized new cells as and when they are needed – sort of like a 3D printer. In medicine they have been dubbed cure-all mini miracles: you'll find them in experimental cancer treatments, dermatology injectable clinics, freeze-dried placenta supplements and state-of-the-art face creams. Their regenerative properties are truly incredible since they contain molecules called growth factors, which stimulate cell growth. But when it comes to skincare, unfortunately you can't always believe the hype.

The FDA issued a warning in 2017 that many stem-cell-related therapies and products readily available on the high street are fraudulent and potentially dangerous. This is because many of the animal- or human-derived stem cells are grown on E. coli bacteria and can produce chemicals as a by-product which, if they aren't purified correctly, can be toxic for the body. Much better are the brands that grow bio-engineered human growth factors on plants, eliminating the toxin risk. There's also an issue with stability of growth factors in cosmetics, and many break down when they're mixed with other chemicals within serums, meaning that by the time you get halfway through your serum, the concentration of growth factors has dramatically decreased.

Also worth knowing is that some **anti-ageing** (see p. 53) creams contain plant stem cell technology and growth factors as opposed to human, which doesn't have to be so rigorously tested before being released onto the market, and often come with some impressive claims that haven't been proven.

Beauty Editor Tip
—

"You can now store tissues grown from your stem cells in stem cell banks, which can then be 'harvested' and used in breast, buttock and penis, yup, augmentations. This is being hailed as the new age of plastic surgery, whereby implants and augment tissues are less likely to be rejected by the body, and come with fewer risks and a quicker downtime than synthetic tissues."

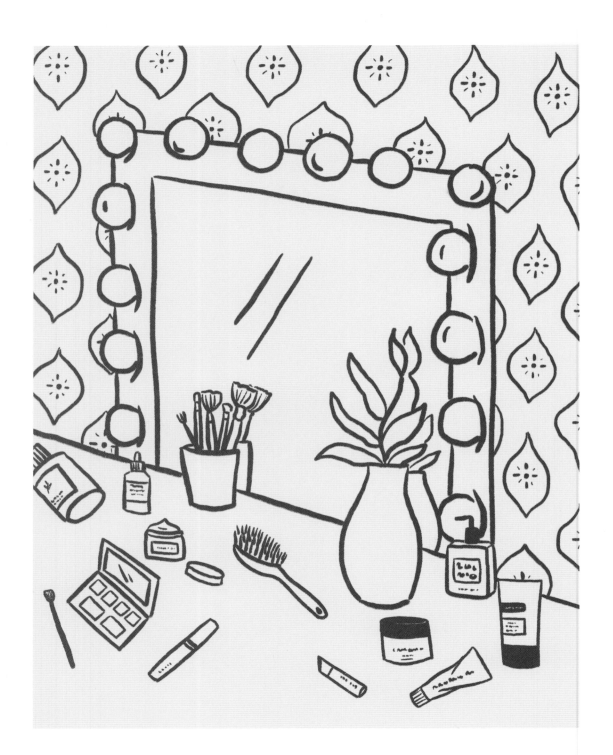

Label Buzzwords

"Anti-ageing"

How healthy is it for our society to use the word "anti-ageing"? This is the question being asked by many body-positive activists out there. Growing older is great, as attested by many who have made it past forty and still love the skin they are in. In 2017, *Allure* decided to ban the word from the pages of their magazine.

"Bi-phase", or "Double-phase"

The salad dressing effect – you know, when oil and vinegar sit separately in the same bottle but mix together when you shake them. You'll find bi-phase formulas in makeup removers and cleansers mostly, but some oil/serum combinations too. In theory they're a great idea, work well and look beautiful on your bathroom shelfie, but beware: for added effect skincare brands often tint them bright candy colours such as mint green, fuchsia and apricot. These colourings are not likely to be natural, so avoid if you have sensitive skin and are trying to cut back on chemicals.

"Cloud Cream"

So-called cloud creams are all about comfort – lightweight, fluffy and moist. But are they any good, or are they just hot air? The texture is a gimmick, so only expect results if the best ingredients are involved.

"Cold-pressed"

Although this sounds like a fad stemming from the green juice movement, cold-pressing plant, seed and nut oils is actually a bona fide method of oil extraction and commonly found in good-quality skincare. The organic material is crushed and pressed, as opposed to distilled, which ensures that the resulting oil is 100% pure and maintains as many of the plant's benefits as possible.

"Choosing ingredients which are gentle and support the healing of the fine skin of the lips is important. I love ingredients like cupuaçu butter (cold-pressed) for its high level of fatty acids and vitamins E and K, and baobab seed oil (cold-pressed) with high levels of vitamin C and as a natural source of calcium, potassium, magnesium and more; it's highly moisturizing, and it's claimed it can reduce fine scarring and fine lines and wrinkles."

Zoë Taylor, Makeup Artist

"Detoxifying", or "Detox"

Your skin goes through its own detoxification processes at night time, and any skincare that assists that is worth trying. But watch out: the word "detox" has been swept up and carried away in a flood of green juice marketing. It's nice to think that using a detox mask will purge away last night's takeaway and transform you into a glowing yoga goddess, but not all "detox" products are as effective as they claim to be. Always consult the label to verify that pore-detoxifying ingredients such as **clays** (see p. 133) and decongestants are actually being used.

"Dramatically"

If I had a pound for every time I read the word "dramatically" on a skincare label, I would be a very rich woman. Please bear in mind that a brand can state that a product dramatically reduces wrinkles without having to prove or quantify that statement. "Dramatic" improvement in skin condition can be achieved in skincare, but not as often as marketing teams would have you believe.

"Fragrance-free"

Whether synthetic or natural, **fragrance** (see p. 30) can be problematic in skincare, as it can be sensitizing. Fragrance-free skincare will minimize the volume of chemicals your skin is subjected to, reducing the risk that it will gradually become sensitized by everyday use. If you can do without fragrance in at least some products, I would recommend it.

"Free-from"

This marketing claim can prefix all manner of perceivably bad ingredients, such as **parabens** (see p. 37) and sulphates. If you see "free-from" on a skincare label, I would recommend flipping the bottle around and checking out the ingredients it does contain.

"I'm not a fan of these marketing terms - 'free-from', 'non-toxic'. From working in the industry every retailer, blogger, brand has a different definition of what this actually means. If brands are true to our word and clear on messaging, then we don't need to be claiming what's *not* in products; let's talk about what *is*!"

Haley Bloom Fitzpatrick,
New Product Developer

"Hydrating"

There's a small technical difference between a hydrator and a moisturizer. Moisturizers help to lock in the water and moisture that is already present in skin, whereas hydrators actively draw moisture into the skin. Hydrating in the evening is important because overnight skin loses a lot of its natural moisture through **transepidermal water loss** (see p. 104). So you really do need to rehydrate before you dehydrate.

"Hypoallergenic"

Similar to "**dermatologically tested**" (see p. 159), "hypoallergenic" is not a legal term. It's a marketing claim that equates to: "we have used ingredients that most people with normal skin won't be allergic to". If you are prone to skin allergies, always patch-test your skincare first.

Beauty Editor Tip
—
"If you are prone to allergies, apply a dab of the product behind your ear and wait twenty-four hours. If your skin is simply irritable, apply it to where your skin is most sensitive. If you want to test whether a product will make you break out, apply a dab between the brows or on the chin, where you are most porous."

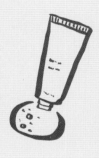

1. Get the Glossary

"Longwear"

"'Longwear' can be tested in customer self-perception studies where participants are asked to assess the wearability of their makeup throughout the day. On the whole, 'longwear' isn't really relevant for skincare, but moisturization testing can be carried out, again, as a customer self-perception questionnaire, or through measured clinical testing."

Haley Bloom Fitzpatrick, New Product Developer

"The phrase 'longwear' makes me laugh a bit. When brands promise 72 hours' wear, I just want to ask: Are you sleeping in it, then? Are you not cleansing your skin? Why are you not washing your face?"

Ateh Jewel, Beauty Journalist

"Magic"

If you believe in magic, then I'm afraid you're reading the wrong book. No single cream or ingredient is magic. Magic will not rid you of wrinkles, and there's no element of hocus pocus that has, to my knowledge, been approved of by FDA or European Medicines Agency regulation. Still, the word "magic" is appropriated by the beauty industry regularly, along with "potions", "elixirs" and the magician-style phrase "gone in a flash!" That said, science aside, there is a genuine rise in spirituality cosmetics if you are that way inclined – everything from chakra sprays to aura oils and crystal-infused creams.

"My cream was actually named by all of the actors, influencers, beauty editors, CEOs, supermodels and starlets who had seen the magic for themselves. I was asked daily for what they called my 'magic cream' because everyone who experienced it knew that Magic Cream was magic skin! I first began mixing this moisturizer to transform models' tired, dull skin during fashion week. It was known as my 'instant miracle turnaround cream' and it rapidly became every celebrity and supermodel's skincare saviour, from the red carpet to on-set and backstage! The iconic cream contains camellia oil, rosehip oil, bio-nymph peptide and hyaluronic acid, instantly flooding the skin with moisture, and it's now world-famous, best-selling and multi-award-winning. I never apply makeup without it!"

Charlotte Tilbury, Makeup Artist and Brand Founder

"Non-comedogenic"

This relates to a skincare product which is formulated so that it won't block your pores. If your skin produces lots of excess sebum or you are prone to **acne** (see p. 127), then non-comedogenic products are a good option for you.

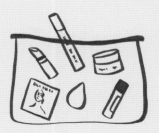

Oil-free

"When I discuss moisturizer specifically, many women are afraid of creams and foundations containing oil, fearing it will be detrimental to their skin, especially if they have concerns regarding their own oiliness. What's tricky to explain is that skincare and good makeup don't add bad, pore-blocking sebum to the skin but fantastic oils that will hydrate, calm, plump up and restore the water/oil barrier in the skin's surface layer. Sometimes this confusion around oil leads men and women to avoid applying oils topically altogether, which can lead to dehydration.

If you layer oil-free, long-wearing foundation on top of thirsty skin, with the best of intentions it can inadvertently create a rather parched, dry, stressed-looking base. Trying to explain to some that their skin is, in fact, dehydrated and would benefit from a little good oil can be really challenging."

Hannah Martin, Makeup Artist

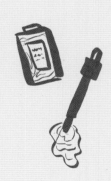

"Oil-free"

It's a common misconception that oil-free skincare is only for oily skin types. It can be used by all skin types and tones. Where you see the label "oil-free", oils will be replaced by synthetic, **water-based** ingredients (see below) that perform the functions of oils (lubricating and moisturizing). This can – not always – reduce the product's capacity to clog pores and cause a skin reaction.

"Pillow Creases"

These are fine lines that seem more exaggerated in the morning. This is in part due to the fact that skin loses a lot of water overnight through **transepidermal water loss** (see p. 104), causing dehydration lines, and in part as a result of the face being pressed and squished into a pillow. Many dermatologists say they can tell which side of your face you sleep on just by looking at the fine lines on your face.

"Probiotic"

This is about good bacteria, but in your face cream as opposed to your Yakult. For some time scientists have agreed that cultivating a good gut biome with probiotics can benefit your skin (bacterial overgrowth in the gut can release too much cortisol, which in turn affects your body's hormone balance, inflammation and skin). In the US, doctors commonly prescribe probiotic skincare to treat **inflammation** (see p. 127) and **acne** (see p. 127).

But now high-street beauty brands have the probiotic bug, using strands of bacteria such as lactobacillus ferment in everything from cleansers to serums in order to reduce skin inflammation and strengthen the skin's natural defence mechanisms. So what's the difference between these products and, say, slapping on some Yeo Valley? Many of the probiotics in moisturizers aren't derived from milk. Some use glycoproteins made in the lab from bifidobacterium, which is much more stable to formulate with and has a longer shelf life. A parting caveat: there is no standardized measurement of the use of probiotics in cosmetics, making it tricky for the consumer to assess the quality of the probiotic and how long it can survive on the skin.

"Purifying"

A non-technical term in cosmetics that is used to describe a wide range of things from **detoxification** of the skin (see p. 53) to deep pore cleansing, it's often employed in association with **charcoal** products (see p. 93).

"Skin Fuel"

This buzzword is often assigned to creams and serums that claim skin-cell-energizing properties. An ingredient one might expect to find in a serum that labels itself as "skin fuel" is **vitamin C** (see p. 39), for example. It's nothing to do with petrol or **petroleum** (although you'll find the latter in plenty of cosmetics; see p. 91).

"Super Foods"

This term relates to **quinoa** (see p. 37), goji berries, **turmeric** (see p. 39), avocado, alfalfa, **kale** (see p. 34), etc. Many of the super foods you'll find in skincare are **adaptogens** (see p. 119), and many are simply a fantastic source of vitamins or omegas. Many more are marketing fads, though, and better off eaten than applied to your skin, where their goodness may not be absorbed as efficiently as via your gut, so do your research.

"Water-based"

Some products use water as a medium to combine formulas and carry ingredients into the skin. Warning! "Water-based" does not necessarily mean "**oil-free**" (see above); these products can still contain a little oil. If you're lucky, they'll contain moisture-loving ingredients such as **hyaluronic acid** (see p. 33) and **glycerin** (see p. 33).

Wake Up to Makeup

Beauty Tips for Brighter Skin

Skincare doesn't stop at moisturizer. I believe that integrating your skincare with your makeup is the fastest (and most long-lasting) route to incredible, glowing skin. Increasingly, the lines between the makeup and skincare categories are blurring into one mega-category: you can now buy eye serums which contain mica and pigments that play the role of a concealer, and mascaras that contain conditioning oils, and fake tans that are blended with essential oils or wrinkle-reducing ingredients. I have designed this chapter to help you understand the "perfecting" functions and ingredients that are now wrapped up into skincare to help make your skin look fresher and brighter.

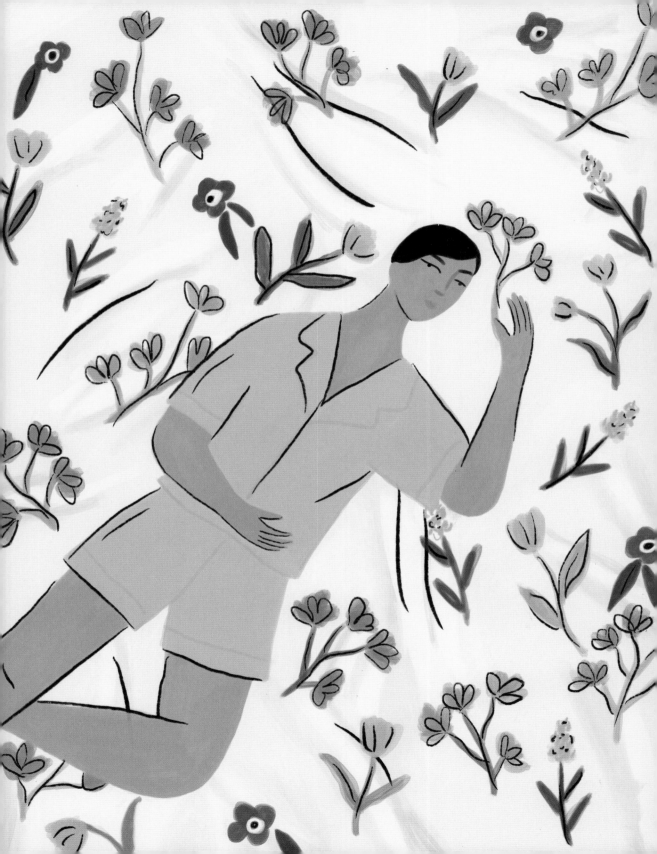

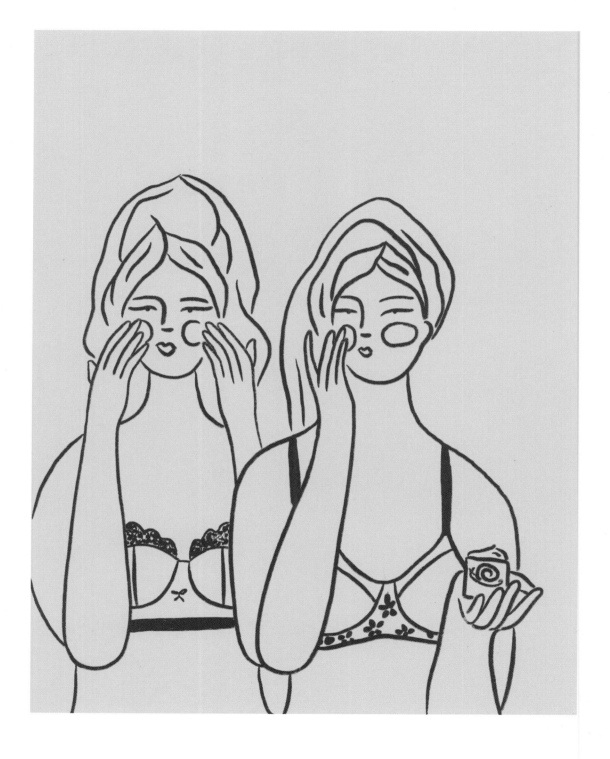

Priming

"The term 'primer' can be a makeup artist's nightmare. While priming the skin before makeup is essential, the availability of primers can lead consumers to believe they are the only thing needed under makeup, when actually makeup primers often don't cater to the skin's needs after cleansing. When I explain that many skin types need a few different products layered beforehand for optimum skin health, comfort and hydration, my suggestions can fall on deaf ears in favour of products that call themselves primers. Negating skincare and simply applying primer - especially dry, silicone-based primers - can promote dry skin and cause foundation to drag, leaving the skin with obvious dehydration lines and patchy foundation where the skin has been thirsty and absorbed whatever moisture it could from the foundation.

To prime skin I'm much more in favour of applying pure squalane, like Indeed Labs Squalane Facial Oil, with a little Kiehl's Ultra Facial Cream on top, and then a balm like Dr. Paw Paw or Elizabeth Arden Eight Hour Cream on any textured skin if necessary. For oily skin, sometimes a light hydrating tonic is all that's needed, with a light water-based moisturizer on the cheeks and an oil-absorbing lotion, like the Estée Lauder Mattifier Shine Control Perfecting Primer, through the T-zone."

Hannah Martin, Makeup Artist

"Breathable"

"Breathable" products, including foundations and nail polishes, are just marketing jazz. Our skin doesn't have lungs and it doesn't need to breathe. If you're worried about your skincare clogging pores and causing spots, then look for the label **non-comedogenic** (see p. 55) instead.

Dimethicone

This popular **silicone** (see p. 38) is used a lot in the makeup space because it's easy to formulate with and provides a satisfying slip to mascaras, lipsticks and eyeshadows. It's made up of relatively large particles that slide over each other easily, and many formulators love it because it's gentle on the skin.

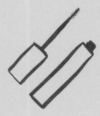

"Dimethicone occurs naturally from silicon dioxide. This silica is then combined with other natural elements, like carbon, oxygen and hydrogen, to form a polymer. Arguably the process it goes through is not natural, but it does stem from a natural ingredient.

It's what gives products their silky smoothness, and can give a mattifying effect and protect from mild skin irritations. There is concern over dimethicone clogging pores, but there's no current published research on this.

I feel it's personal choice whether or not to prefer silicone-free products, but for me I'm not going to rule out using it."

Haley Bloom Fitzpatrick, New Product Developer

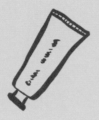

Layering

There are two types of skincare users: those who like to be out the door in five minutes, applying all their skincare in one speedy, multitasking super-serum, and then those who apply their skincare in an extensive sequence of layers, waiting patiently for each application to "sink in" before applying the next. So which is correct? The honest truth is there is no right answer and every beauty editor, brand and facialist will tell you something different. In my opinion, if you follow a simple pattern of cleanse (to remove makeup and dirt), prep (to balance and exfoliate), and nourish (to hydrate, fuel and protect with SPF), then it doesn't matter whether your layers number three or thirty. In the fragrance world,

incidentally, "layering" is also a well-used term, made popular by nose Jo Malone, and involves spraying two or more perfumes over your skin at one time.

"Pore-minimizing"

A beauty myth. The size of your pores is genetic, so unfortunately the idea that they can simply be shrunk on demand is total rubbish. Products that claim to minimize pores either physically block them from view (pore-blurring), using light-diffusing particles and pigments, or contain ingredients that tighten or resurface the top skin layer so that this looks smoother and the pores less obvious.

Velvet

This implies a matte but smooth texture for primers and foundations, and often it denotes a soft-focus or blurring finish. I'm yet to come across a velvet primer that contains actual velvet, but interestingly when Marc Jacobs launched his first mascara (Velvet Noir Major Volume), he was inspired by his mother who used to shave fibres from black velvet ribbon and stick them onto her eyelashes between coats of mascara.

Layering

"I always use a three-part lipcare sequence before any lip colour: scrub to buff off any dry skin, oil to hydrate, and balm to aid in healing. It's essential to treat your lips with the same love and care as you do the rest of the skin on your face."

Zoë Taylor, Makeup Artist

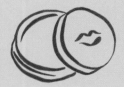

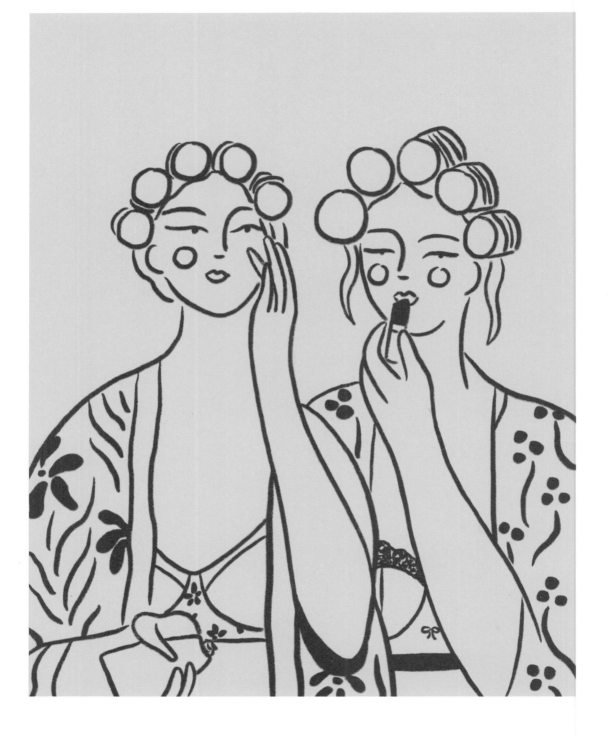

Brightening

Colour-correcting

Tinted cosmetics can be used to disguise unwanted colour undertones in your skin, from blue/green bruises to sallowness and raspberry-coloured broken capillaries. Choose the right tint and you can camouflage anything. Remember learning complementary colours in art class? Well, those same rules apply to colour-correcting. Green neutralizes red, orange masks blue, and lilac warms up yellow.

Beauty Editor Tip
—

"I learned most about colour-correcting while working backstage as a makeup artist, assisting the likes of Charlotte Tilbury and Kay Montano. A lot of time was spent on my hands and knees, hastily covering up bruises on models' shins in the line-up before they hit the runway. Bruises are complicated to eradicate because they contain a spectrum of colours, from yellow to green and purple to blue and black. The golden rule for complete invisibility was to apply colour-corrective concealers in complementary colours with the fingers first, and then to apply a layer of flesh-coloured concealer that matched the skin tone over the top."

Concealer

If you master the art of concealer and maintain a good skincare regime, then in my mind there's no need to waste your hard-earned cash on foundation. As a rule of thumb, look for a creamy, more fluid concealer to paint under the eye area, around the nose and on the chin. Then for blemishes use a drier, pastier concealer and "tickle" it around the area needed with the tip of a small concealer or lip brush.

These are my ride or die concealers:

◇ Laura Mercier Secret Camouflage: use a lip brush and "tickle" this over spots.

◇ Glossier Stretch Concealer: nice and tacky in texture, which makes it easy to apply and great if you love a dewy complexion.

◇ Tom Ford Concealer: the only thing that will eradicate my undereye dark circles.

Beauty Editor Tip
—

"Concealer shouldn't be applied in great blanket washes. It's much more effective to simply conceal the shadows caused by pimples and puffy eyes. The aim is to create an optical illusion that an area that was previously concave and dark is actually a light, flat surface."

Dark Circles

The arch nemesis of every beauty editor. With all the best will and **eye cream** (see p. 45) in the world, sometimes there's no getting rid of the buggers. You see, sometimes they're just hereditary. Other contributing factors may be poor diet, lack of sleep or ironically too much sleep, allergies, stress, eczema, fluid retention (try sleeping with your head elevated on an extra pillow), sagging fat cells, pigmentation issues, excess salt in your diet, and iron deficiency.

Glitter

You'd be forgiven for thinking that glitter was a bit of innocent fun. Far from it. Environmentally speaking, glitter sits in the same irresponsible camp as microbeads and **face wipes** (see p. 103). Made primarily from metal and plastic coatings, glitter particles are not biodegradable, and they're the scourge of our water systems and festival fields. Thankfully, guilt-free glitter is now an option (check out eco rave makeup brands Disco Dust and Eco Glitter Fun), and many festivals are starting to boycott the use of non-sustainable glitter.

Hydroquinone

This controversial **anti-pigmentation** ingredient (see p. 97) is banned in the UK and the EU, but can still be found in face creams in backstreet cosmetic shops, elsewhere around the world, and of course readily on the internet. It works by limiting the amount of pigment (melanin) that the skin produces. There are plenty of studies to say that, when formulated correctly, hydroquinone is a safe and effective ingredient for fading skin pigmentation, but I would advise against it. Firstly, under-the-counter cosmetics can contain any number of unsafe, skin-irritating and potentially hazardous ingredients. Secondly, many products that contain hydroquinone market themselves as skin **"lightening"** (see right) or "bleaching" treatments. Skin bleaching plays into archaic concepts which imply that the paler your skin is, the better it is. There's no place for skin colour prejudice in the beauty industry, so my advice is to say no to hydroquinone.

Kojic Acid

This fungi-derived ingredient is commonly used to brighten the look of skin and fade pigmentation – particularly **acne** scarring (see p. 127), **sun spots** (see p. 95) and skin conditions such as melasma – through the restriction of

melanin production. Is it safe? Yes, absolutely, but always check the label on skin-brightening products for hidden nasties that kojic acid could be combined with, and follow dosage instructions carefully.

Lightening

The controversial term "lightening", or "whitening", is still used by many skincare brands around the world to pertain to **anti-pigmentation** products (see p. 97). Historic prejudice and mixed messaging mean that "whitening" implies it is more beautiful to have lighter skin, which is an unhealthy attitude. All skin tones should be loved and celebrated for what they are. See also **hydroquinone** (left).

Luminizer

This makeup/skincare hybrid (sometimes powder, sometimes liquid) adds a pearlized glow to skin. Most contain light-reflective particles made from **mica** (see p. 69), **glitter** (see p. 65) or **pearl extract** (p. 69), and can be applied all over the face or to zones such as the cheekbones, bridge of the nose and cupid's bow.

Mercury

Absolutely and categorically banned from use in skincare in the UK, US and EU, mercury is still found in some African and Asian **lightening** creams (see above). The FDA lists some scary side effects to mercury when it's used in cosmetics, including kidney damage and depression. The official advice is to avoid unlabelled lightening or whitening creams just in case they contain mercury.

Lightening

"I'm always very suspicious about ingredients that claim to lighten the skin. The whole idea of lightening the skin is dangerous. It goes back to the days of slavery, whereby lighter-skinned slaves were seen as much more valuable than darker-skinned slaves, and this has perpetuated right through history. So there are a lot of people who look at being lighter-skinned as being much more refined and much closer to the Western ideal of beauty. And there are still a lot of people who have that sense that what is beautiful lies in what colour your skin is. I pull brands up on it all the time. I think it's so negative, because what it's saying is that black skin isn't good enough; that you need to lighten it to be acceptable.

Lightening products play on people's insecurities. Hyperpigmentation is something that a lot of darker skin tones deal with, whether through acne scarring or genetics (people want even skin tone whether they're black or white), but I would never ever recommend anyone uses hydroquinone."

Funmi Fetto, British *Vogue* Contributing Beauty Editor

Oxygen

"The epidermis (top renewing layer of the skin) and upper layer of the dermis (supporting deeper layer) receive around 90% of their cellular oxygen supply from diffusion from the atmosphere, so pure oxygen if used very regularly is likely to promote a healthier dermis. This can be seen in medicine in wounds treated with hyperbaric oxygen (much quicker healing time)."

Dr David Jack, Cosmetic Surgeon and Skin Expert

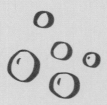

Mica

Mica is a beautiful ingredient, and one of my favourite makeup components. It's a natural silicate mineral – found in the earth – that can be ground up to varying degrees and blended into cosmetics and skincare to add anything from a subtle shimmer to mega-watt shine. You can also find synthetic mica, but both types are biodegradable.

"Non-touring"

The backlash against Kardashian-style, Instagram contouring, "non-touring" is the use of glowy, transparent makeup and skincare – such as glosses, **mineral powder** (see p. 89) and skin balms – to enhance your face shape in a colourless, natural-looking way. I think this phrase was coined by makeup artist Terry Barber, along with "bron-touring" (the same but using bronzer).

Pearl Extract

Crushed or micronized pearls are used to give creams, powders and particularly decadent deodorants a beautiful lumie glow. In Chinese and Ayurvedic medicine, pearls are also ground into supplements to treat **acne** (see p. 127) and promote skin clarity, while in LA you're likely to find a sprinkling of them in nutritional wellness powders. In most cases, freshwater pearls, which naturally contain calcium, magnesium and amino acids, are sterilized first and then ground with some mineral salts to create the extract.

Phthalates

These chemicals are linked to hormone disruption and are now banned from use in skincare in the UK and EU. However, they're still widely and legally used in the US, so keep a beady eye out for them when you're stocking up on your Stateside beauty favourites.

Ring Lights

The YouTuber's best friend, and the beauty photographer's secret weapon. A ring light is a perfect circle of light that attaches to a camera, providing uniform illumination over the subject's face. Flattering as hell, and you can now buy mini battery-powered versions that attach to your smartphone for the perfect selfie. Neat.

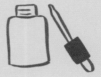

Strobe Cream

A type of pearlized illuminating cream that can be worn alone or mixed in with makeup. The name was coined by MAC, whose best-selling strobe cream is simply brilliant and has since sparked the internet trend for "strobing".

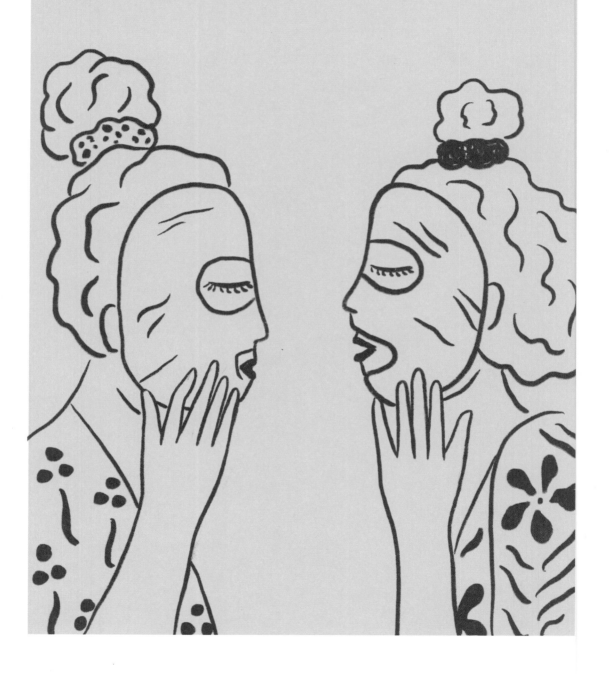

K-Beauty Prep

10-Step Regime

The beautiful "glass skin" (see p. 74) prized by many South Koreans can be attributed to this infamous routine. Move over Clinique's three-step model, K-Beauty recommends ten at least. A standard regime might be: oil cleanser, **water-based cleanser** (see p. 77), exfoliator, **toner** (see p. 104), **essence** (see p. 74), treatment (such as a booster or serum), **sheet mask** (see p. 76), **eye cream** (see p. 45), moisturizer, sun protection. Talk about commitment...

"My daily skincare regime consists of approximately thirteen products. This may seem excessive, but the biggest change in my skin condition came after I started to prescribe to the Asian philosophy of layering skincare. Broadly speaking, this equates to starting your regime with the most fluid texture and building up through to the most viscous formula (usually a moisturizer). I've never looked back. It takes a decent amount of time to execute every morning and evening, but pays boundless dividends."

Mia Collins, Head of Beauty, Harrods

Beauty Editor Tip
—
"Feeling intimidated by so many steps? Many 10-step converts also curate a more manageable 5-step regime for days that require less time spent in the bathroom or, when travelling, less packing space. You can whizz through a single cleanse, essence, treatment, moisturizer and sun protection in no time at all."

Alphabet Creams

Skincare was relatively simple before the invention of alphabet creams; deciphering their uses can sometimes feel as if you're cracking code. In a nutshell, alphabet creams are a fusion of skincare and foundation, but with more **anti-ageing** (see p. 53) functionality than a basic tinted moisturizer. So far there are only **BB** (see below), **CC** (see p. 73), **DD** (see p. 73) and **EE** (see p. 73) creams on the market, but I'm sure it won't be long before ZZ creams fill our bathroom shelfies.

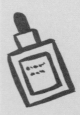

"Baby Skin"

Thankfully this isn't the latest ingredient trend (although **placenta creams** are a thing; see p. 111). It's a phrase used to describe perfectly flawless, poreless skin.

BB Cream

This **alphabet cream** (see above) stands for Blemish Balm or Blemish Base. It's a light cream with an opaque tint to help treat spots while giving a natural-looking coverage. For those of us who are more makeup-minimal, the arrival of cosmetic BB creams came as a godsend. They also contain an **SPF** (see p. 94), making them great for every day, and most will offer moisturizing benefits as well as **anti-ageing** (see p. 53) ingredients.

BB Cream

"While I love the look of BB creams and tinted moisturizers, rarely do I find they can be used alone; they often work best with skincare underneath. BB creams - now widely available and different from the original healing beauty balms made to protect the skin of those who'd had facial surgery and cosmetic peels - vary in their texture, colour and coverage. While I've found some BB creams too dry for some types, others feel more like tinted moisturizers, which I love. I reach for tinted moisturizer - I love the Laura Mercier one - more than I do foundation with clients, as I love the sheer dewiness of the finish, and look to use concealer to add coverage where needed. It's a common misconception that those with acneic skin can't wear tinted moisturizer, but I much prefer to start with a sheer base and then add full-coverage concealer, like the Dermacolor camouflage makeup or Kevyn Aucoin Sensual Skin Enhancer."

Hannah Martin, Makeup Artist

—

"Remember: if you're wearing a cream or base that contains SPF, in order to get full protection from the sun you must apply the product carefully to the entirety of your face. A blob on each cheek won't mean you're fully covered. I have been burned (literally) by this one."

"I love tinted moisturizers as a category, but frustratingly there are limited options for women with darker skin. Traditionally I have had to make it myself by taking my foundation and mixing it with my moisturizer. I think Fenty Beauty has proved that it would sell. I just think people have not been interested in catering to darker skins; they don't see the value in it or the market in it."

Ateh Jewel, Beauty Journalist

CC Cream

This stands for Colour Correcting or Complexion Correcting. Where **BB creams** (see p. 71) target blemishes, CC creams position themselves as correcting redness, sallowness, pigmentation and age spots. In one cream you get a tinted moisturizer texture, heavy-duty concealing capabilities, light-diffusing particles to create dewiness, and an **SPF** (see p. 94). Most promise a natural-looking finish, although not all of them live up to their claims so you may need to try a few to find the right one for you.

Chin Masks

There's no denying these look weird ... Hannibal Lecter weird. Strap one on over your chin and jaw (they hook over each ear) to help tighten loose skin, absorb excess oil, hydrate, and treat blemishes along your jawline. I like to pull mine up over my lips when they're dry too.

"Chok Chok Skin"

A Korean phrase that translates as "moist" or "damp" and is used to describe that glowy, dewy complexion that looks so appealing in advertising campaigns but is harder to pull off IRL. There's a very fine line between greasy shine and Chok Chok shine.

Crystal Iceplant

This is a wonder ingredient for extremely dry or hyper-sensitive skin. The plant – a trendy-looking succulent – grows in particularly arid environments and possesses substances that help it store water.

DD Cream

This stands for Daily Defence or Dynamic Do-all. Things start to get a bit dubious once you pass CC in the **alphabet creams** (see p. 71), and DD creams, while not being technically South Korean, also seem to be an excuse for some brands to reinvent the wheel and market a new multi-purpose tinted serum. But that's just my opinion. As a rule, DD creams act as a defensive shield from environmental aggressors such as UV and pollution, while containing ingredients that will strengthen the skin's moisture barrier.

EE Cream

Too many **alphabet creams** already (see p. 71)? This one stands for Extra Exfoliation and is supposed to help exfoliate dead surface skin cells, brightening your complexion, while also providing sun protection and moisturization. I wouldn't recommend EE creams for everyday use, as a couple of them contain resurfacing ingredients that would irritate or sensitize the skin if used daily. Equally, as a beauty editor, I would recommend exfoliating in the evening, whereas these creams are formulated with **SPF** (see p. 94) for daytime wear. They don't make sense to me!

Egg White

K-Beauty is known for its cutesy sense of humour, and egg white products – including meringue-like foaming cleansers and **pore-minimizing** (see p. 62) masks packaged in egg boxes – are a delectable example of this. Perhaps surprisingly, there is some science behind this eggcellent (sorry) trend. Dermatologists agree that egg white contains plenty of proteins (including skin-tightening albumen) and some **collagen** (see p. 30) for an instant mini-facelift.

Essence

Essentially (ha), essences are simply a South Korean take on a serum. Traditional essences are more lightweight and perhaps less concentrated than serums, and are used early on in the Korean 10-step regime to add an extra layer of nourishment and hydration. But more recently, and since they have been adopted by Western brands, they have increased in potency and thickness, and often have a focus on **cell renewal** (see p. 103) and overnight exfoliation for that "I woke up like this" glow.

Fizzing Face Washes

Fancy a cleanse with a bottle of Perrier? According to K-Beauty, washing your face in carbonated water promotes better skin circulation, clarity and glow. Soaking your face for 15 minutes is supposed to kick-start sluggish cells...

Ginseng

A natural **antioxidant** (see p. 29), **adaptogen** (see p. 119), anti-inflammatory, source of vitamin B and all-round good guy ingredient. There is some interesting research that points to ginseng's ability to inhibit overactive oil glands. Recent studies by the Ginseng Research Centre indicate it could inhibit melanin synthesis and secretion, too.

"Glass Skin"

A K-Beauty skin goal for a complexion that is as clear, smooth, translucent, poreless and gleaming as glass. It's being shiny but in a good way.

Green Tea

A brilliant brew for ageing skin, green tea contains polyphenols and is a potent **antioxidant** (see p. 29). Although the front of the label might boast green tea, the **INCI list** (see p. 168) will cite its Latin name, *Camellia sinesis*.

K-Beauty

"What first drew me to Korean beauty was the packaging, but once we started to import product for my business we discovered that the formulations were light years ahead of what we had previously seen. Korean products are often lightweight and designed to be layered. I don't buy into multiple-step skincare - I like to keep it simple - but equally I don't like heavy formulations. We first brought over some accessories like skin-exfoliating towels and hair velcro - items that made a beauty regime better but added a sense of fun. Korean beauty has really wide psychographics; it transcends age with great design and great formula. The influx of sheet masks is really down to Korean technology.

They also put artisan practices into their development and manufacturing. I remember many years ago my mentor, Japanese makeup artist Shu Uemura, told me that makeup brushes were best made in South Korea. He told me he predicted great things from South Korea in terms of beauty development. I also know that some of the best false eyelash manufacturers are found there. I still use some Korean skincare, from very sophisticated serums like those designed by scientists at the University of Seoul to lip masks for a bit of fun and added moisture."

Millie Kendall MBE, CEO of the British Beauty Council and Co-founder of BeautyMART

Jelly

K-Beauty is partial to this gelatinous texture which liquefies as soon as it comes into contact with the skin. But don't be fooled by its childish appearance; there are plenty of jellies on the market that pack a serious punch in terms of results. One of US Sephora's best-selling products is J.One Jelly Pack, which boasts fragmented **hyaluronic acid** (see p. 33) and a Nobel Prize-winning pollution defence **antioxidant** (see p. 29) called fullerene. Wibble wobble wonderful.

Kaolin Clay

An absorbent natural clay mineral that soaks up excess oil like a sponge, kaolin won't affect the amount of oil your skin produces; it will simply mop it up to leave skin looking more matte and pores less congested. It's also referred to as china clay, hectorite or magnesium silicate. If you have oily skin, it's a great idea to look for a touch-up **mineral powder** that contains kaolin (see p. 89), as well as **clay** masks (see p. 133). This Works Evening Detox Clay Mask is a personal favourite containing kaolin.

Konjac Sponges

Love these: I use them on my face and on my baby. They are made from the konjac potato (or konnyaku) and have been popular in Korea, China and Japan for over a millennium. They are 100% natural and 97% water, as well as being alkaline, which is why they're great for balancing the pH of the skin. Good-quality konjac sponges tick all of the ethical boxes – vegan, cruelty-free, sustainable, etc. – but watch out for

rogue suppliers manufacturing low-quality sponges and selling them on the internet.

Sheet Masks

These face-shaped masks, "infused" with serum, are applied to the skin and then peeled off. They're a huge new sector for the beauty industry: sheet-mask sales grew in the UK by 34% in 2017, and a large part of their success must be attributed to the fact that they are so Instagrammable (search #spaathome for visual evidence). Sheet masks come in paper, gel and fabric-fibre form, with some high-end masks woven from silk or hydro-gel. There are also smaller masks for individual face parts, including **chin** (see p. 73), lips, forehead and eyes, and butterfly masks which are to treat your cheeks and the bridge of your nose. L'Oréal-owned haircare brand Redken has even developed a sheet mask for your tresses. But how do the face masks work? The fabric of the mask forms a physical barrier against your skin, sealing in the **active** ingredients (see p. 49; note these ingredients must be *active* in order to work) and thereby, in theory, making them more efficient. Since sheet masks are relatively new and still considered a little gimmicky, there haven't been many clinical studies to establish just how effective they are on a deeper level. There's not enough real evidence to prove that they will work better than committed application of a good serum, so I personally wouldn't recommend splashing out on the really expensive ones. An interesting new technology, though, is the development of dry sheet masks (amazing for travelling since they are a lot less messy): Charlotte Tilbury's ones are excellent.

"If I have an extra 30 minutes when doing my skincare regime, I spend it on peels and masks. I prefer an acid peel to an abrasive peel. My favourite is the Diamond Glyco peel from Natura Bissé, but I also like the 3-minute peel from La Prairie. I will then follow this with a mask - or two. I love rubber/ modelling masks. My favourite is the Shangpree Gold Premium modelling mask. I'm also a big fan of a sheet mask - particularly when I need a turbo-charged dose of hydration. My favourites include the Colbert MD Illumino anti-ageing brightening mask and 111SKIN's rose gold brightening facial treatment mask, as well as their meso masks for a seriously targeted solution to my naso-labial issues!"

Mia Collins, Head of Beauty, Harrods

Silk Finger Balls

These miniature silk cocoons slip onto your fingertips like tiny pop-socks. Use them to gently exfoliate your skin, decongest pores and improve the appearance of blackheads by massaging them gently in circles around the creases of the nose and chin.

Sleeping Masks

An overnight face mask with a cutesy name. These will contain ingredients that help the skin's natural processes of **cell renewal** (see p. 103) and repair overnight.

Snail Slime

Snails – the French eat them; the Koreans pop them in their face cream. It sounds icky, but reputedly the slime of a snail is a good source of **collagen-boosting** (see p. 30) glycolic acid and hydrating **hyaluronic acid** (see p. 33). The lengths we go to for beauty! But although you may have read about facials which involve the therapist unleashing a couple of the critters on your face, the slime actually has to be extracted ... and if the internet rumours are to be believed, on the whole it's not a humane process. If you're in any doubt, then I advise leaving snail slime out.

Water-based Cleansers

Step two in a traditional Korean **double cleanse** (see p. 45) is usually a water-based or foam cleanser. It's used to remove impurities from the skin, such as dirt and sweat.

Your Morning Routine

1.

Wake up and grab a morning mask (balms work
well for this, and I love This Works' Stress Check
face mask). Apply all over your face and neck.
When we wake, our skin is naturally dehydrated,
so it's a great idea to instantly rehydrate it.

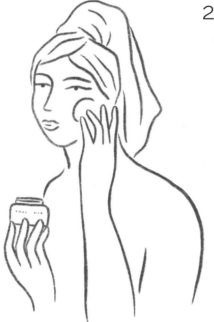

2.

Leave the mask on while you switch on the kettle,
brush your teeth, or do whatever you do in the first
few minutes of your day.

3.

Rinse off at your sink or in the shower.

4.

Big night before and didn't quite get your makeup
off? Cleanse again with a gentle cleanser and warm
muslin cloth.

5.

Next, add some actives to your clean skin. These can take the form of a serum, or a serum and pre-serum/lotion to help the serum absorb better. Apply all over your face and neck. Antioxidants like vitamin C are essential for this step, and preferably something with brightening ingredients like Goldfaden MD's Brightening Elixir.

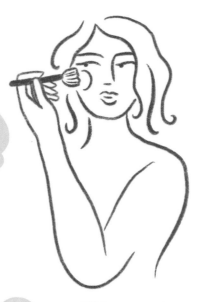

6.

While you wait for the serum to sink in, you can turn your attention to your eyes. Eye patches such as the Elemis Pro-Collagen Hydra-Gel eye masks are easy, quick and affordable, or you can give yourself a gentle eye massage with a refreshing cream if you have time.

7.

Hydrate and protect with a long-lasting moisturizer and a separate SPF or anti-pollution shield.

8.

Finish off your skin with an illuminating primer (nothing too pearlized, but something with glow and colour correction, like Armani Prima's Teint Prima for paler skintones or Becca's Shimmering Skin Perfector in Topaz for darker skintones) before moving on to makeup.

3

On the Go

Skincare Outside the Bathroom

I'm a firm believer that skincare shouldn't just stay in the bathroom. Your bathroom is a safe space – clean, humid and calm – but out there in the big, wide world your skin comes under attack from a huge array of environmental aggressors. Although some products make promises that their benefits will last a full day, it's often out in the real world that you need skincare the most. Whether you're travelling across town to work, or across time zones, or simply across the road, I always recommend taking a mobile, minimized version of your bathroom with you in your makeup bag. Here are the terms and tricks you need to know...

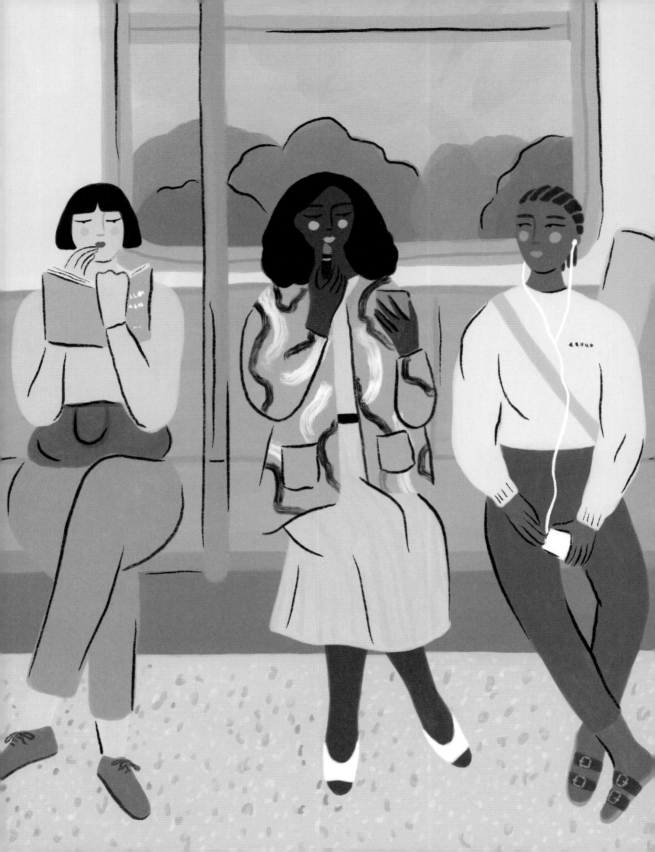

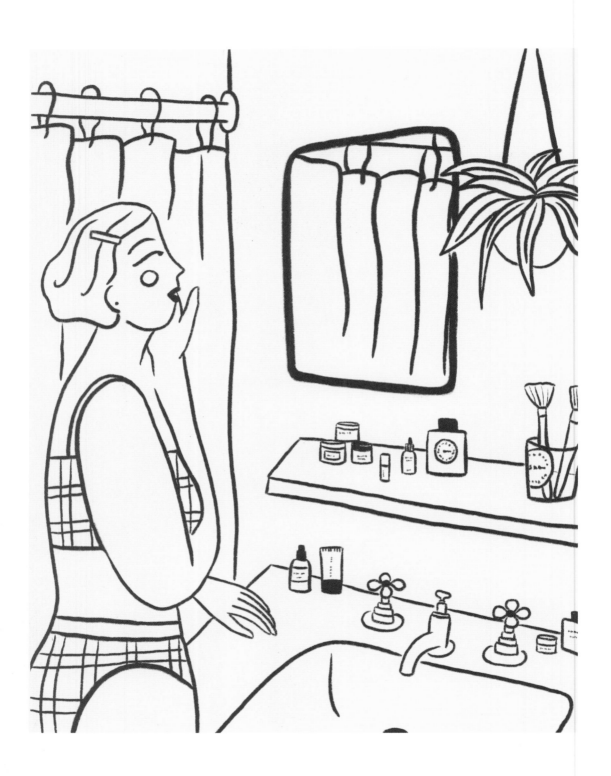

Hand-Luggage Beauty

100 ml

The legal maximum amount of liquid per container that you're allowed to travel with by air in hand luggage … and all must be contained inside a clear standard-issue plastic bag. Lipstick and cream blusher do not need to be in the bag, but gel lip balm does.

Ampoules

Highly concentrated serums of **active** (see p. 49) ingredients with a short shelf life are usually contained within small glass vials with droppers or break-open bottle-necks for single use, aka "mono-dosing". This makes them the perfect travel buddies, and also extra-hygienic.

Capsules

In a similar way to **face wipes** (see p. 103), portable single-use capsules – roughly the size of a supplement, and containing a single dose of oil or serum – are incredibly useful. However, when you think about your daily environmental impact, it's hard to convince yourself that a daily dose of plastic is 100% necessary. Fortunately, there are biodegradable options out there, so look out for these.

Duty Free

The jury's out on whether shopping at Duty Free is actually better value for money. If you compare a lot of the prices in the departure lounge to the ones online, you're likely to find better deals elsewhere. There are savings to be made, though, if you're clever.

Beauty Editor Tip
—
"My golden rules for shopping Duty Free are:

1) Stock up on your regulars. If there's a product you normally buy monthly, even a small saving of £5 will save you £60 a year.
2) Try out travel kits. Duty Free often sandwiches two products together with a small discount, so if you know you need a mascara and an eyeliner then it's a good idea to buy them together in transit. Equally, Duty Free often sells doubles for a cheaper price, which is great, if like me, you like to keep one pot of cream at home and the other in your gym bag/travel washbag.
3) Don't buy your home-grown brands abroad. You will always pay more."

Essential Oils

These are concentrated natural oils extracted from plants, aka Nature's first aid kit. I've placed them in this chapter because, although they're widely used in high-end skincare and fragrance, it's when travelling that I find them the most beneficial. When inhaled, essential oils can have an aromatherapeutic effect on the body. On a very basic level, essential oil molecules trigger a chemical reaction in the limbic system of the brain when they come into contact with the cilia – the hair-like antennae in your nostrils. The limbic system is the same part that deals with emotion and memory, and studies have proven that essential oils can have an effect on your mood. There are essential oils like **lavender** (see p. 108) that calm you down from stressful situations, and others such as **camomile** (see p. 107) that help you sleep. On the flip side, others can rev you up: I like to inhale some **ginger** (see p. 31) before an important meeting, for example. Other oils, such as **frankincense** (see p. 107), can equip you with a sense of tranquility in challenging situations. Remember, synthetic fragrances won't stimulate the brain in the same way, therefore any bath oil that claims to help you sleep but only contains synthetic lavender is pulling your leg.

Hand Cream

If you're going to take the time to regularly massage cream into your hands, for goodness' sake make sure it's going to do something! Hands have very specific concerns and therefore require some targeted ingredients – a generic moisture cream just won't cut the mustard. Hands are constantly exposed to the elements and so would benefit from **SPF** (see p. 94) to defend against UV damage and hydrating **hyaluronic acid** (see p. 33) to combat dryness from air-conditioning. Hands also get knocked about and so soothing, calming ingredients such as **arnica** (see p. 119) will help reduce swelling and bruising, while **vitamin E** (see p. 39) will help reduce the appearance of small scars.

Beauty Editor Tip
—
"Get into the habit of rubbing the backs of your hands with any excess serum after you've applied it to your face. It's the reason I don't buy hand creams."

Makeup Fixers

These sprays are divided into two categories: the type that fixes your makeup in place and then the type that "finishes" it, adding a dewy glow. The former usually employs alcohol, which evaporates from the skin, pulling moisture away along with it; this mattifies makeup in the process and helps it last longer. The latter uses **hydrating** ingredients (see p. 54) to moisten makeup and to keep it looking fresh. NB Alcohol in skincare is very drying so, if your skin is naturally dry, try to avoid makeup fixers with an alcohol base, or check that the product also has hydrating ingredients on the **INCI list** (see p. 168).

Masks on the Move

Sheet masks (both dry and wet; see p. 76) are the nomad's best beauty friend. Travelling, especially by air, can be very stressful and dehydrating for your skin, so masking can help replenish some of the lost nutrients and natural moisturizing factors. If you're too embarrassed to wear a sheet mask in public, try a **jelly** (see p. 76) mask, which is a bit less conspicuous.

"My absolutely favourite Chanel skincare product has to be Sublimage Essential Revitalising Mask. It is a miracle in a bottle. This beautiful mask makes skin look utterly incredible. I use it as a prep on celebrities and models, as skin looks so luminous, hydrated and plump afterwards."

Zoë Taylor, Makeup Artist

Travel Minis

Is there anything more satisfying than stocking up on travel minis in the airport? But it sure as hell ain't cheap. Muji makes fantastic travel containers that you can decant your regular products into if you're on a budget. Also if you do like to splash out on a travel mini or two, remember that you don't have to buy them last minute at the airport. Non-departures brands such as Percy & Reed, This Works and Elemis all do brilliant travel-sized heroes.

Essential Oils

"When I arrived at *Vogue*, despite being inundated with a million products I tended to find the simple aromatherapeutic ones with high-quality ingredients worked better than most commercial cosmetics. I still drink hot lemon, eucalyptus and ginger when I'm ill, rather than a pharmaceutical option, and I like nothing better than to put drops of essential oil in my bath to energize, relax or ward against colds and flu."

Kathy Phillips, ex-British *Vogue* Beauty Director, Author and Aromatherapy Expert

Your In-Flight Brief

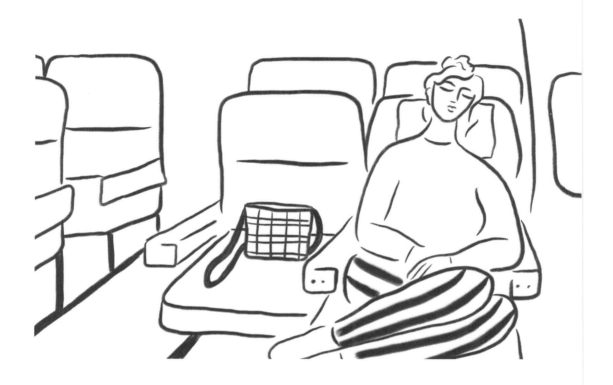

1.

First things first, take off all your makeup. Getting on a flight with clean skin is the best thing you can do to help you get off the flight looking radiant. Use a biodegradable cleansing towel or head to the bathroom to wash away any makeup traces and the pollutant particles that your skin picked up on the way to the airport.

2.

Next, apply an anti-inflammatory serum containing adaptogens (a gel will feel nice and cooling) to your face, neck and chest.

3.

Keep a time check and, using a facial mist with hydrating ingredients such as hyaluronic acid, keep your skin topped up with moisture on the hour, every hour.

4.

As you land, reach for a lip balm and an illuminating primer, giving your cheeks and jawline a good massage to stimulate blood flow, and start readying your appearance for your welcome party in arrivals.

5.

If flying solo, I always use a Colbert MD Illumino sheet mask in the taxi from the airport. Its plumping and brightening effect is miraculous after a long-haul flight, and always ensures I need to use less makeup afterwards because my skin just looks better.

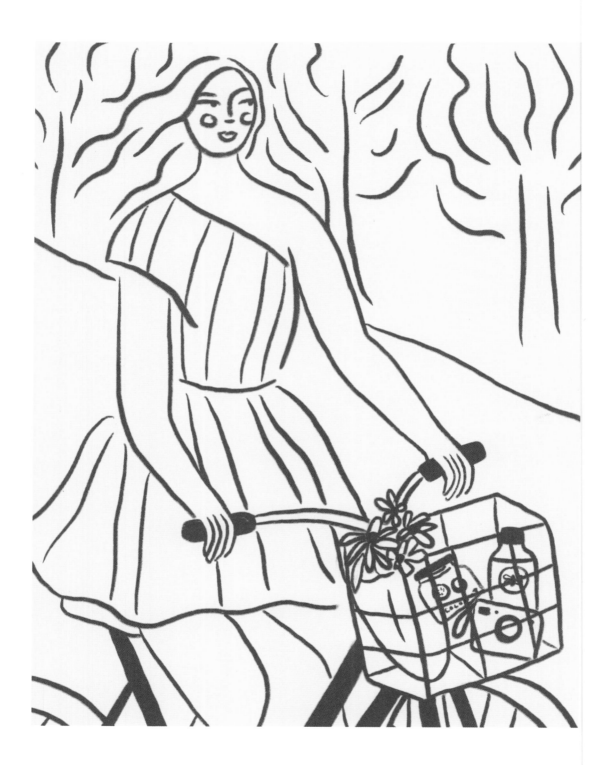

On-the-Go Ingredients to Know

Beeswax

The base for many on-the-go skin balms, beeswax naturally creates a comfy, waterproof barrier over the skin, locking in moisture, which is why it's so popular for lip balms. Like all natural products, it does have a propensity to cause irritation to some people, so if your lips are feeling worse after a day of lip balm application it's worth considering whether the beeswax base is the cause. Its Latin name, so you can spot it on the **INCI list** (see p. 168), is *Cera alba*. It's definitely not considered vegan, in case you were wondering.

Coconut Oil

Coconut oil (or coconut butter) is extracted from the inner white flesh of the coconut. It takes over twenty coconuts to produce 1kg of oil. There are plenty of reasons why beauty aficionados go nuts for the stuff. It's rich in fatty acids and **antioxidants** (see p. 29), which means it's deeply **hydrating** (see p. 54) and protective, respectively. It's also one of the rare natural oils that is classified as non-irritating. There are some internet myths that you can use coconut oil as suncream on holiday, but while most studies agree that it does contain a natural sun protection factor in vitro (as does **olive oil**; see p. 91), the US National Library of Medicine puts it only at about SPF7, which isn't enough to rely on as your only form of protection, so don't risk it. On the other hand, have you tried shaving with coconut oil? Or using it as eye makeup remover? It's also a good vegan lip balm option.

Jojoba

A lovely, natural, **fragrance-free** oil (see p. 54; **coconut** and **beeswax** both have a fragrance – see above) jojoba is an effective skin-soother because it has a similar consistency to the sebum in our skin and contains plenty of fatty acids and **antioxidants** (see p. 29). It's also light and non-greasy-feeling. Safe for vegans.

Lanolin

Unlike other lip-balm bases that act as moisture barriers, lanolin can itself deeply moisturize because its molecular structure mimics the lipids already within the skin. It's, rather bizarrely, secreted from the sebaceous glands of sheep. It therefore may not count as **vegan** (see p. 14), but most would agree it's certainly **cruelty-free** (see p. 15) since it's removed from the wool that has already been shorn from the sheep.

Mineral Powder

Mineral powders stepped into the spotlight in the late 1970s, then peaked in popularity again when Bare Minerals launched in 1995. When packing hand luggage, mineral foundation powders, blushers and bronzers are a brilliant alternative to liquids. But beware: just because they use the word "mineral" on the label doesn't mean they are all good. They may still contain ingredients that are seen as dodgy, such as **talc** (see p. 91) or **parabens** (see p. 37).

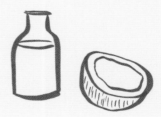

On the Go

"I always keep a clear plastic makeup bag packed with my travel skincare kit ready to go (Susanne Kaufmann does a great one), instead of using one of the bags from the airport. They're sturdier, usually a little bigger so I can sneak in more of my skincare routine, and nicer on the eye, plus it means I've always got my skincare essentials at the ready, instead of last-minute panic-packing face wipes - a skincare no no! Also solid cleansing balms/bar soaps, etc. are a great way to avoid the liquid limit. I love not wearing any makeup to the airport - granted, it's not my best look, but it means I can try any new skincare products in Duty Free and then pass the time on a long-haul flight doing a full facial, or, for a shorter flight, some eye masks. Institut Esthederm are my go-to. Instead of spending loads of money on holiday minis, I invest in some clear mini plastic bottles and decant my serum/moisturizer/cleanser/sun cream into these each time I fly. They're under 100 ml so they fit in hand luggage, and it's much better for the planet to have something that's reusable.…

For day to day, on my way to work every morning, I apply lip balm (I love Dr Sam Bunting's Flawless Lip or La Mer's lip balm), and use the excess on my finger to brush up my brows and give them some nourishment at the same time. I'm often guilty of doing my makeup on the tube, too, but mascara and eyeliner on a moving train can be messy. My trick is to cross your legs and lean the elbow you're holding the mascara or eyeliner in on your knee to steady it. That way, when the train moves, your hand should stay put."

George Driver, Digital Beauty Editor, ELLE UK

Olive Oil

The most basic of beauty products and an ingredient that has been used for thousands of years with relatively few hiccups along the way, since it has a very low reaction rate – and if that's not a testimonial then I'm not sure what is. Olive oil contains dryness-quenching fatty acids and some **antioxidant** (see p. 29) benefits. When mixed with other skincare ingredients it provides a smooth, glide-on texture to the formula. See **coconut oil** (p. 89) with regards to olive oil containing a small amount of natural **SPF** (see p. 94). Its Latin name, so you can spot it on the **INCI list** (see p. 168), is *Olea europaea*.

Paba

Or, if you prefer a scientific tongue-twister: para-aminobenzoic acid. An active ingredient that used to be a common find in sun lotion, it got some bad press for causing skin reactions in the 1990s and so is rarely used in modern formulations. Check your ingredients label just in case.

Petrolatum, or Petroleum Jelly

'When applied to the skin, this occlusive semi-solid gel forms a barrier, preventing any water loss (though personally I don't find it helps to moisturize my lips). Petrolatum is 100% natural (made from hydrocarbons) and has to be a certain level of purity to qualify as "cosmetic grade". Vaseline Petroleum Jelly labels itself as "triple purified". Petrolatum is **non-comedogenic** (see p. 55) and so, before you start pointing the finger, it's probably not the ingredient in your moisturizer that is giving you spots. It is, however, a by-product of the oil industry, so perhaps should not be on your beauty line-up if you're looking to make more eco decisions.

Talc

A powdery natural mineral filler for absorbent skincare products, foundations and face powders, talc is relatively unpopular in UK formulating for two reasons: 1) its white and chalky finish now looks outdated next to today's dewy textures, and 2) there have been several lawsuits connecting talcum powder to cancer, although the supporting evidence is so far weak and the FDA still considers it a safe ingredient in the US. If you're looking for a trouble-free alternative, rice starch is a great option. Spot talc on the **INCI list** (see p. 168) as talcum powder or cosmetic talc.

Triclocarbon, Triclosan

Everything you wash down the sink has a consequence. These two synthetic ingredients are a good example. Although they are legally formulated with, as antibacterials and preservatives in soaps and toothpastes, they are environmentally persistent – in other words, they never actually disintegrate and so get stuck in our water systems eternally – and may be associated with hormone disruption in humans and animals.

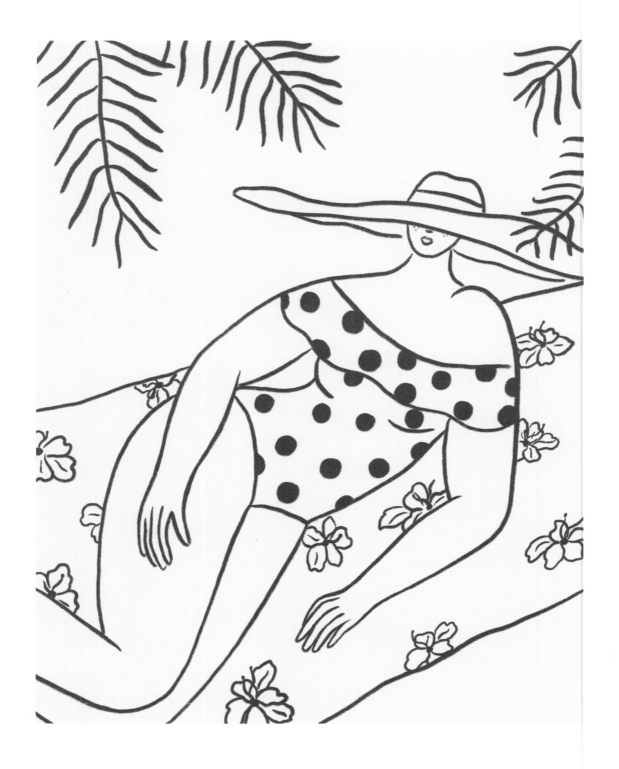

Skin Protection

Activated Charcoal

Aka beauty's dirty little secret. Great for acne-prone skin, the best quality is made from charred bamboo. In order to absorb toxins and excess sebum from your skin, the charcoal has to be treated with an extremely high heat (over 1000°C). Good-quality activated charcoal products (and, as with all trend-led ingredients, there will always be poorly made products to avoid) contain the minerals zinc and copper, **vitamins E, C**, D, B1, B2 and B12 (see p. 39), and folic acid, which makes them naturally anti-inflammatory and antibacterial.

Barrier Repair

Your skin has an outermost layer of cells called the stratum corneum or lipid barrier, designed to be the gatekeeper to the lower levels. It's composed of about 15–20 layers of flattened cells, but it can be weakened through dehydration or exposure to pollution, UV or irritants, compromising overall skin health. Sensitive, reactive skin often has a weakened barrier function. Ingredients that strengthen and repair the barrier are, for example, **niacinamide** (see p. 37), **hyaluronic acid** (see p. 33) and **cica** (see p. 30).

Chemical Sunscreen

These products are sometimes referred to as synthetic sunscreens, organic sunscreens or chemical absorbers, which makes things complicated. Essentially, chemical sunscreens are organic compounds (organic, as in made from carbon in a lab, not the kind that is grown on a farm in Somerset) which create chemical reactions within the skin to transform UV rays into heat that can then be released externally. There are over twenty-five different types of these chemical/synthetic sunscreens, and some names you might spot on the **INCI list** (see p. 168) are octinoxate, oxybenzone, octisalate and avobenzone. Cosmetically, those with darker skin tones might prefer to use this type of sunscreen (as opposed to **mineral sunscreens**; below), as they tend not to leave a chalky white stain on the skin on application or when encountering water or sweat. The golden beauty editor rule is: apply, reapply, and wear a hat. The sun is the number one cause of skin ageing.

Glycation

This is the bombardment of our skin cells by excess sugar molecules, aka sugar-induced ageing. That's right, as if you didn't have enough to worry about, what with free radicals and UV-pollution-induced wrinkles, now you have to guard against sugar too. Studies have shown that people with higher blood sugar counts tend to look older than they actually are. Something to think about when you order that next hot chocolate...

Malachite

This wonderful natural mineral has free-radical-fighting abilities, since it's rich in the trace mineral copper. Malachite is currently enjoying a renaissance (it was big in cosmetics in Ancient Egypt), both in **anti-pollution** skincare (see p. 97) and in crystal-healing-based skincare.

Mineral Sunscreen

There are two types of mineral sunscreen: **titanium dioxide** and **zinc oxide** (see p. 95). These ingredients work by sitting on the surface layers of the skin and acting like mirrors to deflect the sun's harmful UV rays, bouncing them off again. I like to imagine them as tiny little soldiers with shiny shields held in formation up to the sun. One of the disadvantages to these two sunblocks is that some of the larger-particle versions can appear white or chalky on the skin.

Moringa

While sunscreen is the only way to actually protect your skin from the sun, natural ingredients such as moringa oil, thanks to its high **antioxidant** (see p. 29) content (specifically **vitamins A** and **E**; see pp. 113 and 39), can help your skin cells fight against photodamage and reduce **inflammation** (see p. 127) caused by this. If you're into naturals, this stellar ingredient is well worth looking out for.

Nanoparticles

To combat the white glare that physical sunblock provides on the skin (think Baywatch nose stripes in the 1980s), formulators now use both **zinc oxide** and **titanium dioxide** nanoparticles (see opposite) in sunscreen. Essentially, these are much smaller-sized molecules and do not reflect visible light; instead, they reflect non-visible light, such as UV rays, without appearing white on the skin. A note of caution: try not to inhale spray sunscreens containing zinc oxide or titanium dioxide.

Natural Sunscreen Alternatives

The only natural sunscreen alternatives I would ever recommend are wearing a hat and staying out of the sun. Unfortunately, while some natural ingredients (e.g. **coconut oil**, see p. 89; the beta-carotene in carrot seed oil; and raspberry seed oil) do have natural sun-protecting factors, these are only in minimal amounts and cannot stand up against the protection you would get from a **chemical** or **mineral sunscreen** (see p. 93). Just don't risk it.

"It's hard to say what a natural sunscreen is by definition, because there are no standards for this term. Generally speaking, though, natural sunscreens tend to perform consistently less effectively than their chemical counterparts, especially when it comes to UVB protection. Also, many sunscreens, even with 'natural' ingredients, can disturb coral reefs, since a lot of what we wear is washed into the sea when bathing, etc. It's a difficult area, since there is no standardization of protection."

Shabir Daya, Co-founder of Victoria Health

Physical Sunscreen

Another name for **mineral sunscreen** (see p. 93). Confused yet?

SPF

This stands for Sun Protection Factor, and it's the measure of how long a product will protect your skin cells from damage when they are exposed to **UVB** rays (see p. 95). If your skin starts to burn without sunscreen on after 3 minutes, then suncream with SPF factor 30 will keep you protected for 90 minutes (3 x 30) before you begin to burn. SPF100 is apparently on its way...

Beauty Editor Tip
—
Three great facial sunscreens for darker skin tones:

1) Terry UV Base Sunscreen Cream
2) Paula's Choice Sunscreen SPF50 for Face and Body
3) Skinceuticals Ultra Facial Defense SPF50

Sun Spots

These brown and white pigmentation marks develop from time spent in the sun. 90% of visible signs of ageing are due to sun damage. In Asia, women are more concerned about sun spots than they are wrinkles, which is why South Korean **anti-ageing** (see p. 53) imports often contain ingredients that tackle pigmentation, such as **vitamin C** (see p. 39) and **niacinamide** (see p. 37).

Titanium Dioxide

One of the two types of **mineral sunscreen** (see p. 93). You can spot it on the **INCI list** (see p. 168) as titanium white, CI 77891 or Pigment White 6.

UVA

These long-wave ultraviolet rays from the sun penetrate deep into the dermis of the skin. It used to be thought that only **UVB** rays (see p. 95) were a danger to our skin, but increasing research into the effects of UVA rays shows them to be just as troubling and to play a major role in photo-ageing and skin cancer by damaging the skin cells called keratinocytes in the epidermis (the layer of the skin where most cancers occur). UVA is the light that is primarily used in high-street tanning booths and, according to the Skin Cancer Foundation, the high-pressure sun lamps used in salons emit doses of UVA as much as twelve times that of the sun. Not surprisingly, if you use a tanning salon regularly, you are 2.5 times more likely to develop skin carcinoma than a non-user. Also, first exposure to tanning beds in youth increases melanoma risk by 75%. Some ingredients to look out for that protect skin against UVA rays are avobenzone, dioxybenzone and oxybenzone.

UVB

These short-wave ultraviolet rays from the sun tend to burn the superficial layers of the skin, causing long-term damage, including contributing to the development of skin cancer by damaging the skin's cellular DNA. **SPF** (see p. 94) protects skin from these rays for limited amounts of time. Staying out of the sun is the only fail-safe protection.

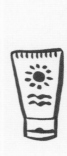

Zinc Oxide

One of the two types of **mineral sunscreen** (see p. 93).

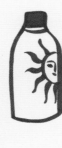

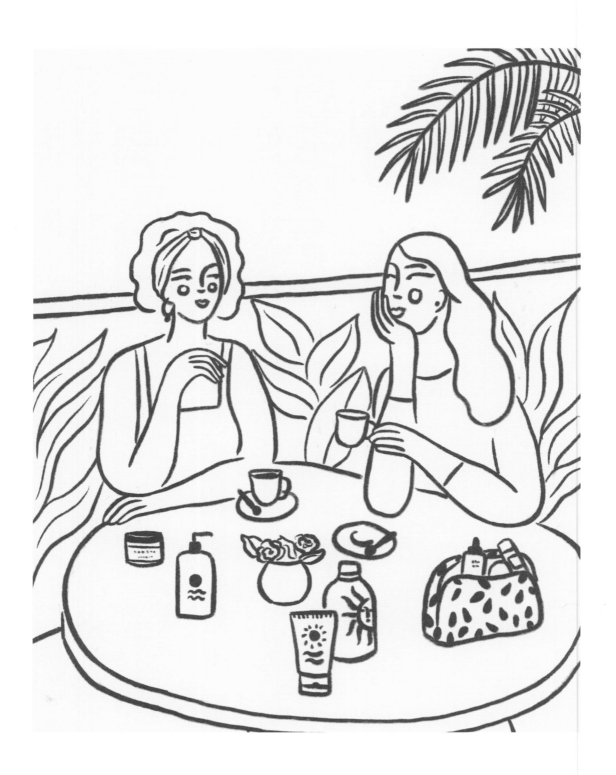

On-the-Go Beauty Speak

Anti-pigmentation

This term covers skincare that counters a whole host of pigment issues, from age spots and **sun spots** (see p. 95) to hyperpigmentation, melasma and **acne** scarring (see p. 127). Since it's such a broad umbrella term, it's important to check the label for which ingredients are included. See, for example, **niacinamide** (p. 37), **hydroquinone** (p. 66) and **vitamin C** (p. 39).

"I think it's important to take a multi-faceted approach to pigmentation in black skin, as what works for some people may not work as well for others. Not only must the depth of the pigmentation in the skin be considered, and treatments designed accordingly, but it must be kept in mind that darker skin types, particularly mixed skin types, can react to any sort of irritation from treatments by *increasing* pigmentation.

In my opinion, gentle beginnings is always the key, getting the skin used to particular products and techniques, then building up as the skin is desensitized. Starting from superficial treatments - peels such as mandelic and lactic acid, together with vitamin C-based products - can be effective in lifting superficial pigmentation and stimulating reduction in scar tissue. However, these are generally treatments that will need to be repeated multiple times, over several months, to really notice significant changes."

Dr David Jack, Cosmetic Surgeon and Skin Expert

Anti-pollution

This is one of the most important beauty buzzwords to emerge this decade, and a category that promises to grow and grow as pollution levels rise and rise. A CNN headline in 2019 even declared that "the latest weapon against pollution is skincare". Anti-pollution skincare guards against "polluaging", where microscopic pollution particles squeeze themselves like cat burglars into the gaps between cell walls and disintegrate to cause free-radical damage to the skin structure. Pollution contributes to fine lines, clogged pores, urban acne and skin sensitization. It can also make skin conditions such as eczema worse. As the saying goes, the best offence is a good defence, so using a product that contains free-radical-fighting **antioxidants** (see p. 29) daily if you live in an urban area is a good idea; for example, Oskia CityLife Anti-Pollution Facial Mist. Equally, using a cleanser or **essence** (see p. 74) with decongestive properties after a day in the city is well worth it, too.

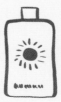

Cellulite Cream

If **cellulite** (see p. 139) creams could actually make you skinny, then trust me they would be a lot more expensive. I am hugely distrusting of any cream that promises to help you shed dress sizes or lose weight, because this category is prone to mismarketing, and that constitutes emotional hijacking. No cream will remove fat cells from your body; for that you'll need to take a trip to your dermatologist (see **Kybella** and **CoolSculpting**; pp. 144 and 140). To be fair, most cellulite creams on the market only claim that they "help improve the appearance of cellulite", which is a different thing altogether. Both **caffeine** (see p. 29) and **retinol** (see p. 112) are found in most cellulite creams worth their salt. Caffeine acts like a diuretic, flushing water from the area and firming it up temporarily, and retinol refines the surface of the skin, making it appear smoother and more supple.

Inflammaging

This is skin ageing caused by chronic, persistent **inflammation** (see p. 127). Stress, sun exposure and pollution can all contribute to inflammaging.

Microbiome

This is the eco-system or "'me'co-system" of micro-organisms that live across the surface of your skin. That's right, your face is crawling with them. But before you start feeling itchy, it's important to understand that most are completely harmless, and some even perform vital functions for us. Since our skin is our interface with the outside world, it's important to culture and support the microbiome; see **probiotic** skincare (p. 56).

Pollenution

The double whammy of city smog and a high pollen count is a perfect storm, manifesting itself in congested pores, urban acne and red, puffy skin. According to the University of Worcester's National Pollen and Aerobiology Research Unit, pollution can make pollen grains more fragile, which causes them to explode and dial up the amount of allergen in the air.

Beauty Editor Tip
—

"If you're prone to hayfever and live in the city, it's a wise idea to pollenution-proof your skin from first thing in the morning. You can do this in a couple of ways: firstly by hydrating the skin so that the lipid barrier functions well throughout the day, and secondly by using a serum with both anti-inflammatories to calm any hayfever-induced swelling and antioxidants to form a defensive barrier against pollution particles."

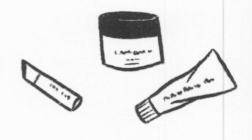

Inflammaging

"Cold water is really important with regards to removing inflammation and the whole ageing process of the body. What cold showers do is stimulate the vagus nerve, which interacts with your main organs … and your biggest living organ is your skin. So when you switch on the vagus nerve it resets your endochrine system, it resets your immune system, it resets your gut as well. And all these things have an effect on the skin. So just by simply cold showering you're going to reset your ageing process. I also like to freeze small doses of my serum in ice cube trays and apply them frozen."

Nichola Joss, Facialist

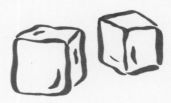

The Night Shift

Skincare Before Bedtime

Something special happens to your skin when you sleep. While your mind switches off, your skin cells become an exciting hive of activity. They whirr into action, repairing damage that's been done to them in the day, dealing with toxins that have worked their way into your system, and regenerating and growing new parts. This is why just before you go to bed is a great time to apply skincare, because by the time it's soaked in and you've nodded off, your skin cells can make use of all the ingredients in all the functions that they're required to carry out that night. You know the phrase "get your beauty sleep"? Well, that's a real thing. In the following section, I have listed some of the best ingredients for night-time use, as well as some nightmare ones to avoid.

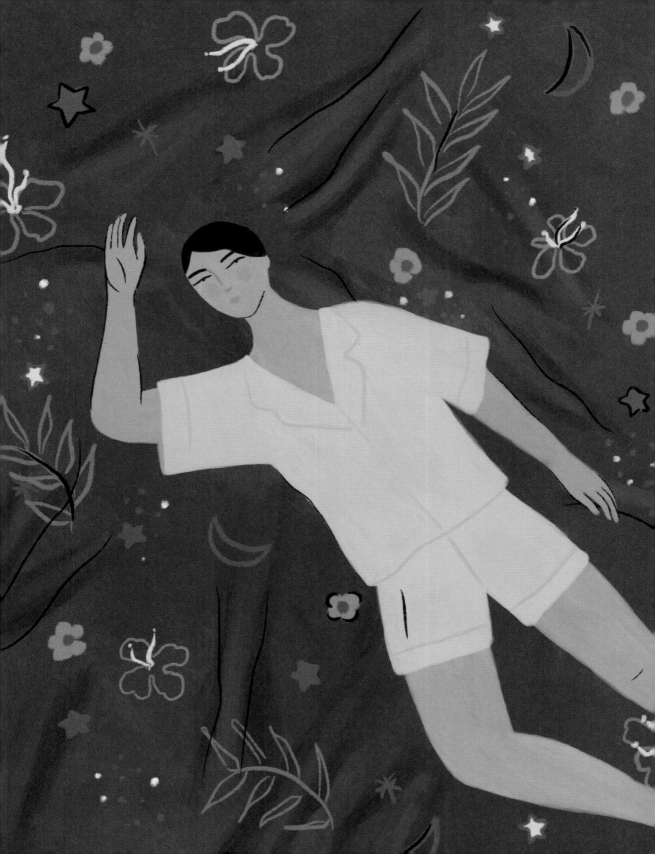

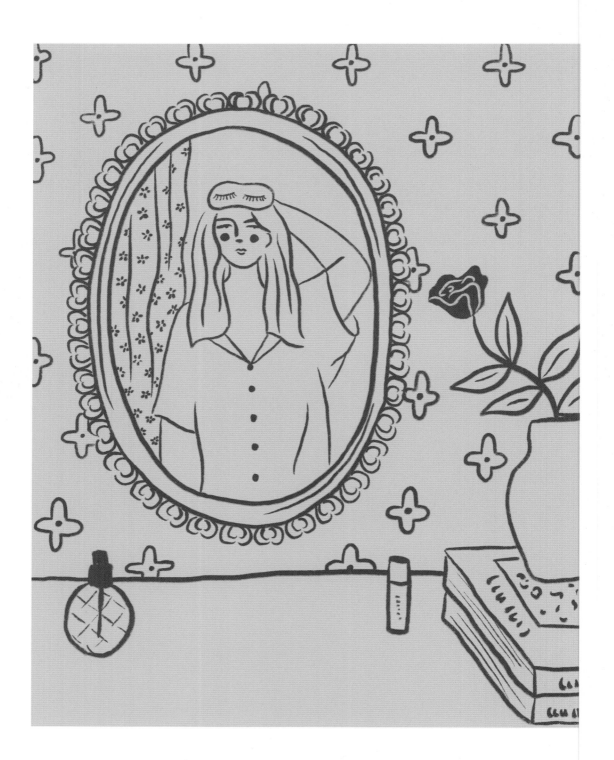

Evening Prep

Cell Renewal

The process of shedding old and dead cells from the surface layer of your skin, to be replaced by new cells underneath, is a gradual process (a cycle that lasts about twenty-one days) but it's important for skin that looks fresh and healthy. As we age, cell renewal slows right down, which is why beyond your late twenties you should look for ingredients that boost your cell turnover by speeding it up or supporting it, such as **fruit enzymes** (see p. 107), **retinoids** (see p. 113) or **hydroxy acids** (see p. 107).

Eye Cream at Night

If you choose to use an **eye cream** (see p. 45), you may want to think about swapping in a different one from day to night, just as you would your moisturizer. I wouldn't, for example, recommend an eye cream that contains **SPF** (see p. 94) to be used round the clock, since there's no need for sun protection at night. Skin cells naturally repair themselves overnight, so picking ingredients such as **lavender** (see p. 108) and squalene, which will support that repair, is important.

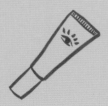

Face Wipes

There's a long way to go in the "banishing face wipes from our supermarket shelves" crusade. The trouble is they are just so convenient for "lazy cleansing" and travel packing. If the environmental impact of using face wipes doesn't trouble you (Water UK has disclosed that wet wipes make up 93% of the matter blocking national sewers because they don't biodegrade), then perhaps the knowledge that most don't actually clean your face efficiently will dissuade you. Essentially you're just pushing dirt around your face, since most wipes will leave residue including daily grime and makeup on your skin, making you more prone to spots than when you use a regular cleanser. If you really can't face binning the wipes, then eco versions do exist: Neal's Yard make a biodegradable organic cotton wipe, and RMS Beauty make theirs with **coconut oil** (see p. 89) and 100% compostable rayon.

Fake Tan

Self-tanning products have come a long way since the "you've-been-Tango'd" days of yore. In fact, products from brands such as Tan-Luxe (their tanning water is the only product I have used successfully without streaks), St. Tropez and James Read have really revolutionized the world of tanning. There are now tanning **mists** (see p. 42), tanning makeup powders, overnight tanning face masks and, of course, tanning **sheet masks** (see p. 76). My favourites are spritz-on tanning waters, which are refreshing to apply and simultaneously treat the skin with **anti-ageing** (see p. 53) ingredients. Traditionally self-tans use the tanning agent DHA (dihydroxyacetone – the one that smells like rich tea biscuits, though nowadays it can be formulated with a much softer smell), which works by reacting with the amino acids in the top layer of the skin and developing a shade of brown.

Hot Water

Although a piping hot flannel may feel lovely to cleanse with at the end of a long day, it may be sensitizing your skin. The American Academy of Dermatology advises using lukewarm water instead.

Makeup Remover

The rumours are true: taking your makeup off before bed is one of the most important skincare steps and pivotal to good skin. With the exception of **face wipes** (see p. 103), most cleansing methods — from **double cleansing** (see p. 45) to **coconut oil** cleansing (see p. 89) to **micellar water** (see p. 41) — will help lift the surface layer of dirt and grime from your pores, enabling the skin to better repair and detox itself while you sleep. Avoid foaming cleansers that contain skin-irritating **sodium lauryl sulphate** (see p. 39).

Resurfacers

These products or ingredients chemically help speed up the process of **cell renewal** (see p. 103) and/or physically lift off the surface layer of dead skin cells. Always check the label if you're planning to use a resurfacer every day: some are particularly strong and designed to be used only once or twice a week, whereas others have a weaker concentration that is specifically for daily use.

TEWL

This stands for transepidermal water loss — the evaporation or diffusion of water through the epidermis, which peaks overnight, leaving skin dehydrated come morning. All the more reason to hydrate every evening with a moisturizing night cream or serum.

Toner

Over the years toners have boasted astringent properties to dry out oily skin, or included pH-balancing ingredients, or simply been an extra layer of moisturization. The important thing is that they should provide a good base layer after cleansing for the rest of your skincare: so hydration and skin-restoring ingredients. Avoid toners with drying alcohol and synthetic **fragrance** (see p. 30).

Evening Prep

"My evening cleansing routine is pretty simple. I usually use coconut oil on recyclable cotton pads (or RMS make amazing coconut oil wipes) to take my eye makeup off, just because I find it's hydrating, so I'm not stripping the skin around my eye area with something drying.

Then I'll use two pumps of Goldfaden MD Pure Start cleanser with cool water, which helps with any redness I have and to calm my skin down, closing any open pores I might have too. I love cleansing with cold water. I don't wash my face with hot water ever, as I don't like what it does to my skin."

Lisa Goldfaden, Co-founder of Goldfaden MD

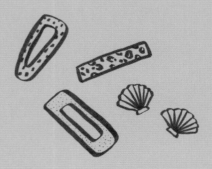

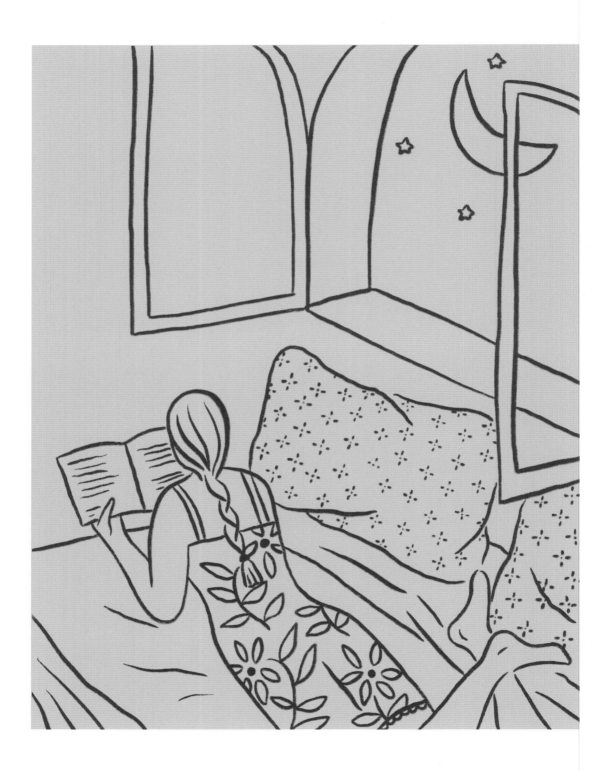

Nocturnal Ingredients

Astaxanthin

A super-**antioxidant** (see p. 29). And when I say super, I mean super-duper. It's often dubbed "the King of Carotinoids". According to Dr Shabir Daya of Victoria Health, astaxanthin is sixty-five times more powerful than **vitamin C** (see p. 39), fifty-four times more powerful than beta-carotene, and fifteen times more powerful than **vitamin E** (see p. 39). In supplement form, there are many clinical studies to prove that astaxanthin can help improve skin texture and firmness in just a couple of weeks. You'll find it in plenty of antioxidant serums on the market, although most studies are based on taking it in supplement form. There is also some evidence to say that it reduces the effectiveness of **retinol** (see p. 112) and so shouldn't be combined with this.

Camomile

Most famous for its soporific effect when drunk as a tea, this flower is also a winner in skincare. As an extract, it has anti-inflammatory, skin-soothing properties as well as being a natural antiseptic. As an **essential oil** (see p. 83) in aromatherapy, it's used as a natural anti-anxiety ingredient, helping to calm the mind and promote sleep. Spot it on the **INCI list** (see p. 168) also as chamomile, Roman chamomile or *Chamaemelum nobile*.

Frankincense

The most incredible **essential oil** (see p. 83) when used in aromatherapy, frankincense has a grounding effect that helps the user pause, breathe and feel revitalized in a calm way. It's a great oil to scent your home or bath tub with. In skincare I'm afraid it's not so useful, with no clinical trials proving it as a majorly beneficial **anti-ageing** (see p. 53) ingredient. It can also be a bit sensitizing to skin.

Fruit Enzymes

Employed in exfoliators to help remove the top layer of dead cells from your face and body, fruit enzymes reveal a smoother, clearer skin texture underneath and are a great help in managing frequently blocked pores. They work by speeding up the breakdown of the keratin protein that holds the dead cells together. They are gentler than many chemical peels and exfoliators that you'll find at a dermatologist, since they only remove dead cells and not living ones as well. As a result, they can be used in your daily skincare regime. You may see them referred to as "multi-fruit enzymes" or "multi-fruit extracts", and common fruits used are papaya, pineapple and blueberry.

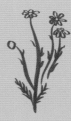

Hydroxy Acids

This is an umbrella term for a collection of whizz-kid exfoliators, namely AHA, BHA, LHA and **PHA** (see p. 108), the common link being that they are all molecules that contain carboxylic acid. Similar to **fruit enzymes** (see p. 107), they help speed up the natural shedding of dead surface cells, revealing the smoother skin underneath and helping to unclog cluttered pores in the process. They have plenty of unique properties as well as similarities: for example, AHAs are great at reducing the visible signs of photodamage, while BHA (there is only one, **salicylic acid**; see p. 129) is oil-soluble and can work inside the pores to help unclog them. LHAs are keratolytic, which means they help lift off the top layer of dead skin cells. PHAs tend to be gentler on sensitive skin, since they have a larger molecule size and are less likely to sting or tingle on application. Can you use them all at once? There's nothing stopping you – and it wouldn't be hard, since they are found abundantly in everything from **scrubs** (see p. 43) to **essences** (see p. 74) and cleansers – but it can feel like a bit of an assault on the skin: a better idea is to alternate them on different days. The great thing about them is that they work fast: you can see the beautifying results of a hydroxy acid overnight.

Lavandin Oil

Known as poor man's lavender because it's cheaper than fancy Provençal lavender, lavandin is extracted from a hybrid plant that produces a much higher volume of the oil, making it cheaper to manufacture with, but you'd be unwise to dismiss it because of that. There are some really interesting (and apparently paradoxical) studies now linking lavandin to stress reduction and reduction of nervous energy, but also invigorating the body when tired.

Lavender

The queen of calm. As an **essential oil** (see p. 83), lavender has been proven in numerous clinical studies to promote a sense of calm within the nervous system, decrease mental anxiety, lower the heart rate and blood pressure, and contribute to a better, more restorative night's sleep (sleep is a beauty category in its own right). The best lavender in the world is Provençal lavender. See also p. 123 for lavender's skin-soothing properties.

Beauty Editor Tip
—
"If you don't like scenting your pillow with lavender oil because you're not a fan of the smell, why not try applying a few drops to the soles of your feet – an aromatherapy hotspot."

PHA

This stands for polyhydroxy acid – a variety of **hydroxy acid** (see p. 107) that's worth knowing about if you have sensitive skin, as it's known to be similar to but gentler than AHAs. This is because PHA is made up of larger molecules, which can't penetrate the skin as deeply. Not many products formulate with it, but since its much-written-about usage in Glossier's Solution exfoliator (see p. 176), it's bound to increase in popularity, which is no bad thing.

Water

As much as it may make sense, our skin does not drink H2O. Topically, as an ingredient, water won't make great strides with **hydrating** skin (see p. 54), whereas ingredients such as **hyaluronic acid** (see p. 33) and plant extracts will. So why is "aqua" so often listed as the first ingredient on the **INCI list** (see p. 168)? Well, it's frequently included as a solvent, which means it helps to hug all the other, more **active** ingredients (see p. 49) together, or it can help to "deliver" other hydrating ingredients into the dermis. It's a safe bet because it's cheap and rarely aggravates the skin. Nowadays we're all so obsessed with water, though, you may well want to know where the aqua comes from. It's hard to tell whether you're covering your skin in pH-balancing mineral water or good old-fashioned tap water unless it's stated on the label, but if it does concern you then look for brands like Skyn Iceland, which uses glacial **Icelandic water** (see p. 33), or La Roche Posay, which uses thermal spring water.

Lavandin Oil

"People don't tend to realize how many and how varied the types of lavender are. But the difference between lavandin and other varieties of lavender is vital, as they have opposite characteristics. For instance, 'true' lavender is relaxing, sedative and antiseptic, while lavandin - a hybrid or clone of the original, with a different chemical profile, sometimes referred to as *Lavande batarde* - is energizing, even stimulating. It's important, then, not to use lavandin for sleeplessness (where you need *Lavandula angustifolia*), but it is invaluable as a mosquito repellent, and it's the one to put in with your sweaters to repel moths. It can be used to clear your head if you have a cold, due to its high camphor constituent, but it's not the right choice for a soothing bath before bedtime.

Lavandin is generally grown at lower altitudes than the best 'true' lavender and is not considered to be as fragrant. It's also less expensive and tends to be used for household products, soaps and detergents, whereas varieties like *angustifolia* and especially Maillette lavender are chosen for 'haute parfumerie' due to their superior aroma. René-Maurice Gattefossé, a scientist and pioneering aromatherapist in the 1920s, extolled the virtues of high-altitude lavender from Provence as having the best and most therapeutic properties."

Kathy Phillips, ex-British *Vogue* Beauty Director, Author and Aromatherapy Expert

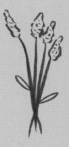

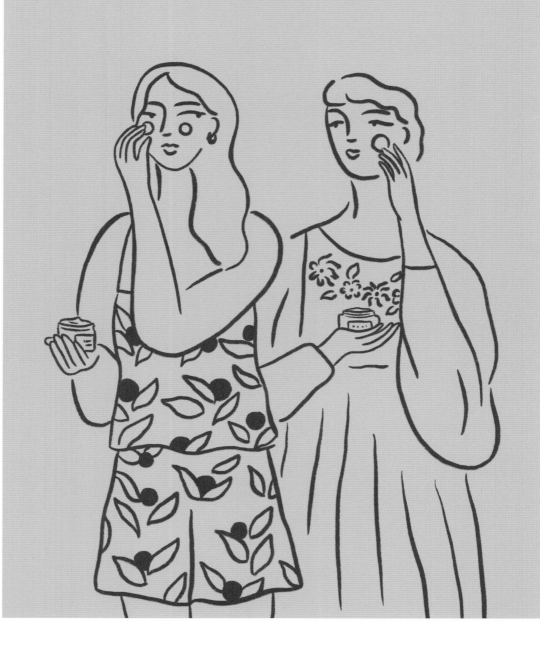

Overnight Anti–Agers

Bakuchiol

Pronounced *buh-KOO-chee-all*, this ingredient is being heralded by beauty bloggers and naturals fans as "the natural alternative to **retinol**" (see p. 112). I have a problem with this statement because some retinols *are* natural. What people mean to say is that bakuchiol is a plant-based ingredient. It increases cell turnover in a similar way to retinol, but does so much less aggressively since it also has a soothing, calming effect on the skin. It's completely safe for use during pregnancy.

Coenzyme Q10

If you always wondered what the Q10 of Nivea Q10 stood for, allow me to enlighten you: Q10 – vitamin Q or ubiquinone – is an enzyme that is found naturally in our skin and has an antioxidative effect on skin cells. The levels of Q10 in our skin are depleted by the environment (pollutions, UV, etc.) and topping up levels topically has been proven to show some improvement in skin's appearance. Over in Asia it's big news, but it's also a firm favourite in French pharmacy brands.

Elastin

This is the protein that keeps our skin bouncy, allowing all the connective tissues within our bodies to stretch and spring back like an elastic band. Depressingly, stocks of this wonderful springy stuff get depleted by exposure to sunlight and the ageing process, leaving skin to sag and droop until eventually the body stops making it altogether. Sorry to be the bearer of even further bad news but, unlike other youthful components that naturally occur in our skin such as **hyaluronic acid** (see p. 33), elastin is useless when applied in a cream or serum.

Ferulic Acid

This brilliant **antioxidant** (see p. 29) is found in lots of food and plant sources – from flaxseed to **ginseng** (see p. 74), and even cooked sweetcorn – and helps repair and protect from the damage done by environmental pollutants. It's an excellent addition to your serum if you're an urbanite. It's also reported to increase the efficiency of **vitamins C** and **E** (see p. 39). SkinCeuticals C E Ferulic is a beauty editor favourite.

Peptides

If skin proteins such as keratin and **elastin** (see left) were buildings, then peptides would be their bricks – kind of a big deal when it comes to skin structure. Similar to **antioxidants** (see p. 29), there are plenty to choose from – some from natural sources and others that are synthetic, created or tweaked in laboratories to get them to perform better. So what do they do? That totally depends on what type of peptide, but in general they do things like reinforce the skin's natural barrier and increase skin firmness, helping to restore and renew skin overnight. Spot different peptides in **INCI lists** (see p. 168), prefixed by the word "palmitoyl".

Placenta Creams

Yes, these are a thing. Why? Well, placentas contain an incredible amount of **stem cells** (see p. 51), human growth factors, and obviously all the fabulous nutrients to help build a baby. Placenta creams are also obviously quite controversial. Firstly because there isn't enough research to categorically say that magi-mixing a placenta and applying it to your skin will help reduce wrinkles (although there are plenty of creams and facials on the market that promise it does), and secondly because there are some (also unresearched) concerns over the level of **oestrogen** (see p. 134) they contain. They are also of course not vegan-friendly. Most you'll find in facials or face creams are from sheep, but there are companies that will, if you so desire it, scoop up your placenta post-partum and turn it into a face cream. Having given birth, I can tell you that after 48 hours of labour you couldn't pay me to go anywhere near my placenta but, hey, each to their own...

Quercetin

This is a good **antioxidant** (see p. 29), which helps to fight off the ageing effects of free radicals and to repair damaged cells.

Retinoids

Derivatives of **retinol** (see below) are called retinoids. I'll list some here in order of strength, starting with the strongest: retinoic acid, retinaldehyde, retinol and **retinyl palmitate** (see right). Starting on a retinoid feels a little like joining a secret cult: you have to be initiated with a low level of the stuff in order to progress on to the secret revelations of the top potency. It requires commitment and lots of cash, but the results are addictively good (unlike most cults, they're backed by science); before you know it you'll find yourself hooked for the long term. Skin looks noticeably smoother and fresher even after a week's use. I'd argue for this reason that retinoids are even more addictive than **Botox** (see p. 153).

Retinol

Another name for **vitamin A** (see right). See also **retinoids** (above).

Retinyl Palmitate

A fusion of two good **anti-ageing** (see p. 53) ingredients – retinol (see left) and fatty acid palmitic acid – this is a great starter ingredient for those wanting to dip their toe into hardcore anti-ageing skincare for the first time. It's not expensive on the high street (hurrah!), and it's more gentle on the skin than other retinol derivatives.

Vitamin A

One of the most popular **anti-ageing** (see p. 53) and anti-acne treatments in the business, mainly because it's one of the only ones that is clinically proven. You may have spotted it in the skincare aisle going by another name, **retinol** (see left). In layman's terms, it works by speeding up the lifecycle of skin cells and by preventing the breakdown of **collagen** (see p. 30) deep within the dermis, reducing the formation of deep wrinkles. You'll notice that many products advertise a percentage of retinol: if you have sensitive skin and are new to retinol, then you might want to start with something nice and low, for example 0.25% or 0.025% if you have a darker skin tone. The highest percentage of retinol you can get without needing a prescription is 2%. Skincare brands often boast about their high percentage, but more important is to look at the other ingredients paired with it: neat retinol is fantastic, but skin needs a diverse cocktail of ingredients to function at its best. A final point: if you are buying a vitamin A/retinol product, be careful to check the packaging. Anything that lets in air will "spoil" the ingredient, thus diminishing its effectiveness – a tube is best.

Beauty Editor Tip
—
"If you use a retinol eye cream or a retinol moisturizer around the eye area, make sure to avoid wax when you're getting your eyebrows shaped. One bad experience left me with the top layer of skin stripped off and scabs along my brow bone for weeks. Not attractive."

Retinoids

"Retinoids have been a game changer for my acne-prone skin. I was nervous in the beginning. There are so many horror stories online, but a trusted dermatologist talked me through the facts (getting expert advice is my number one rule), and I've been using a prescription retinoid called Treclin for over a year now.

I use it three to four times a week in the evening on cleansed, dry skin. I apply a few dots on my forehead, cheeks and chin, and massage in. When possible I wait fifteen minutes and then apply a La Roche Posay Sensitive Riche moisturizer. The waiting time is to avoid diluting the retinoid.

Would I recommend it? A big, resounding yes. Remember, retinoids are a bit like divas. They're only going to work if you give them your full attention and use them properly. They're not something you should use half-heartedly."

Sarah Jossel, Beauty Director, *Sunday Times Style*
#thebeautyboss

Your Night-Time Routine

1.

As soon as you get home, even if it's only 5pm, remove everything with a double cleanse: one to take the makeup off, and two to clean your skin.

2.

Spend time massaging through your cleanse process because when you massage you open up the lymphatic system and allow toxins and pollution that are sitting in the skin but also in the muscle tissue to be drained out, so you're removing deep-rooted pollution as well.

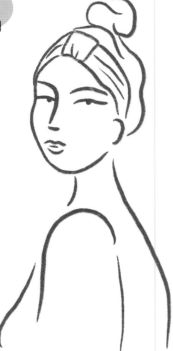

3.

Make the experience relaxing. Choose cleansers with a soothing, anxiety-relieving scent to help you mentally unwind from your day.

4.

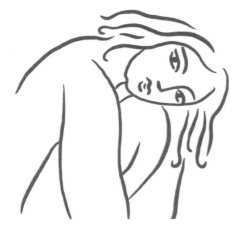

Next, spritz your toner or whatever facial product you're putting on to refresh your skin or rebalance it.

5.

Your active ingredients should go on at this point. This is so that any actives that need time to purify pores or exfoliate can get to work before you use a moisturizer or oil to lock things into your skin.

6.

Enjoy your evening, eat your dinner, watch your favourite Netflix show.

7.

Just before bed time you can use a wonderfully rich night cream or an oil. The reason you might put an oil on at night as your last layer of skincare is because this will drop deep into the skin, locking in the active ingredients you put on four or five hours earlier.

SOS

Skincare Saviours

Sunburn, peeling, breakouts, bacne, liver spots, rashes, cracked lips and sore spots... Bad skin happens to good people. We've all been there. But if you're having a skincare crisis, the worst thing you can do is panic and throw the kitchen sink at it. Aggravated skin doesn't take much to become even more aggravated (and inflammation leads to premature skin ageing), so my best advice if you want to save face is to avoid piling needless ingredients into the mix that could make the situation worse. Take a step away from the bathroom sink and think: "What single ingredient or technique might help put out the flames of this miniature Vesuvius that has erupted on my face?" If you need some level-headed inspiration, then read on for my list of SOS skincare.

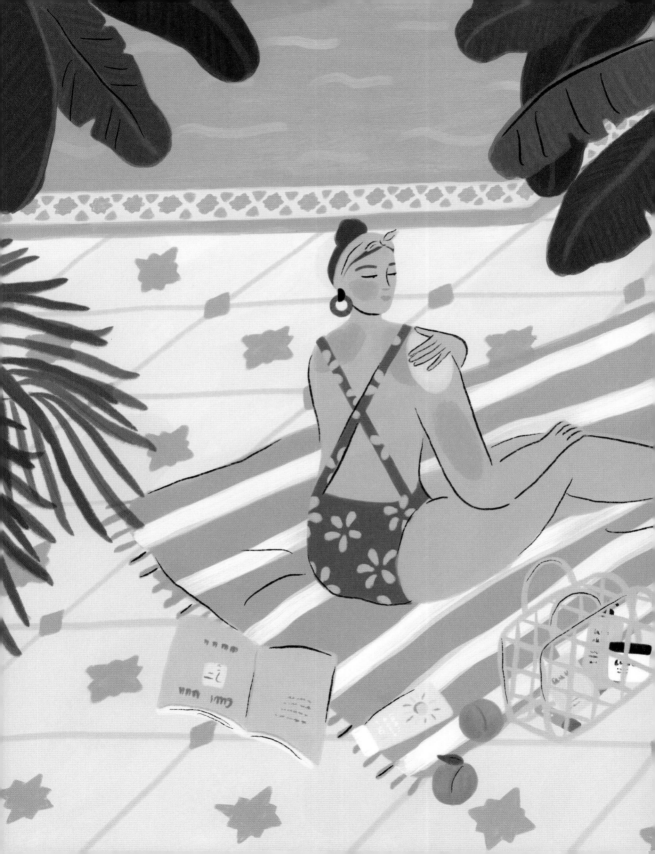

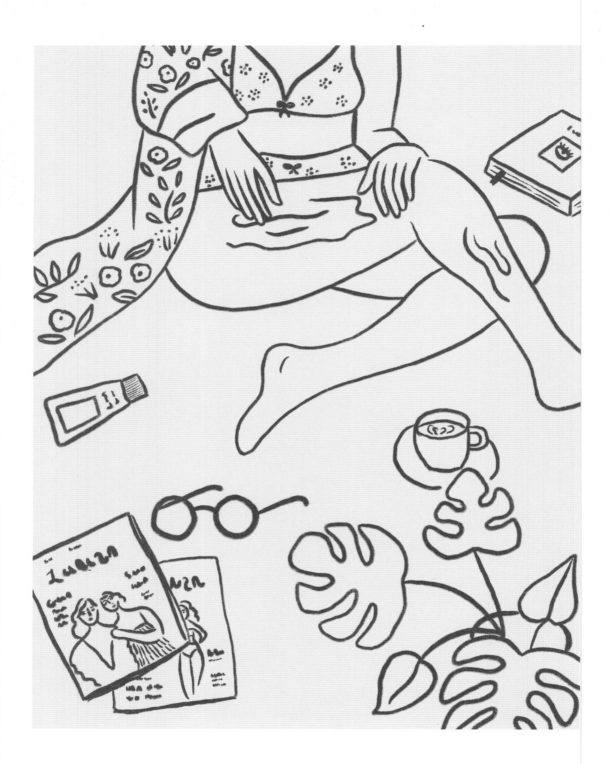

Ingredient Fixers

Adaptogens

Want skin that's more zen? Adaptogens are helpful herbs – including ashwagandha and **turmeric** (see p. 39) – which manage the stress hormones released from the adrenal glands. In skincare, they are often loaded with **antioxidants** (see p. 29) and anti-inflammatories.

Arnica

The bruise buster. Arnica is obviously brilliant in body creams to help soothe damaged skin and fade away bruises. A little-known fact is that it's also brilliant in **concealers** (see p. 65) and **eye creams** (see p. 45) for reducing the swelling and puffiness from undereye bags.

Camphor

An ancient herbal **essential oil** (see p. 83) similar to menthol, camphor is used for mild pain or itching relief. It has that recognizable "deep-freeze" cooling effect on skin, which works by stimulating the nerve endings and increasing blood flow to a particular area, thereby distracting from any discomfort. Unfortunately camphor is an ingredient that comes with a high risk of irritating the skin, but nonetheless there are some great natural products on the market that contain it, if you don't seem to be affected by sensitization – in particular, yoga gels and muscle rubs, which I love to apply just before or after a session on the mat. Just make sure you wash it off your hands and don't get it anywhere near your eyes: the sting is unbearable! If you fancy the refrigerator effect without the risk, then look for products that contain gently cooling **cucumber** extract (see right) or **aloe vera** (see p. 123).

★

Cucumber

Will cucumber slices actually help reduce puffy eyes, or are they better off in a salad? Cucumber extract is mildly soothing, but the real benefit is more likely to come from storing cucumber in the fridge and applying it to the skin cold. The cold will help reduce swelling and puffiness.

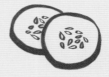

Repair Cream

This is a handy addition to your skincare arsenal, particularly for occasions when skin feels sensitive or is over-exposed to environmental menaces such as aeroplane air-con, commuter grime or central heating. Repair cream is designed to support and rebuild the skin's natural barrier and should contain a number of naturally moisturizing **active** ingredients (see p. 49). The best ones, in my opinion, are French pharmacy brands and unscented so as not to risk sensitizing the skin even further, such as Mixa Repair cream.

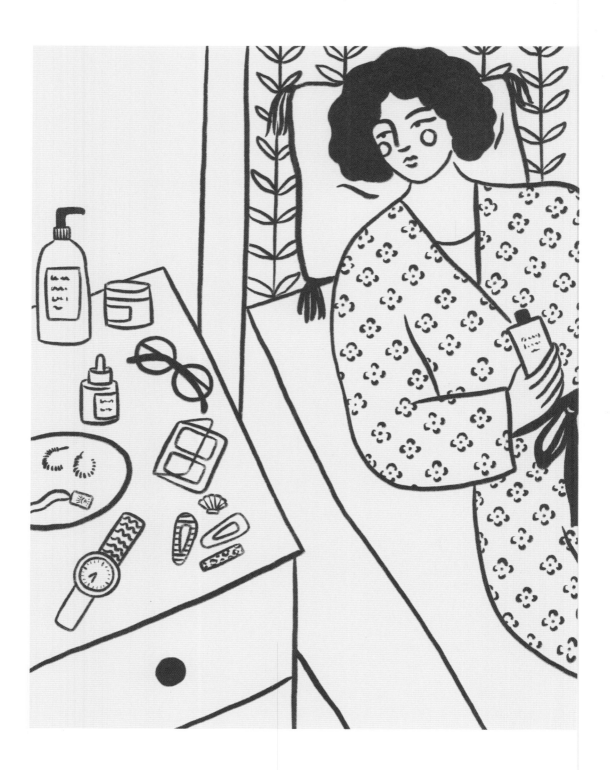

Calming and Soothing

Almond Oil

A calming natural oil that is rich in fatty acids and natural moisturizing factors. Almond oil has zero **fragrance** (see p. 30) and so won't trigger any adverse skin reactions, making it an excellent choice in a skin crisis such as cracked heels or post-holiday **peeling** (see p. 123).

Vitamin E

See p. 39 for information on this skin-regenerating and repairing powerhouse. NB Most internet sources will tell you to apply the stuff neat to scars to help reduce their appearance, but studies suggest this is a myth, and in some cases it can actually make them worse.

Calamine Lotion

An old-school treatment for insect bites and sunburn. On application, the calamine evaporates from the skin, resulting in a cooling effect. Calamine lotions often contain **zinc oxide** (see p. 95) or carbonate as well, which add to this soothing feeling and also have antiseptic properties.

Ice

Frozen H2O is a potent secret weapon. The humble ice cube (wrapped in gauze) is a superior sunburn soother, eyebag de-puffer, circulation and blood-flow booster, and post-workout or injury compress to reduce swelling. You can pimp your ice tray with all sorts of frozen beauty goodies. Uber makeup artist Lisa Eldridge once told me that she likes to freeze cubes of **green tea** (see p. 74) to slide over and brighten a tired complexion early in the morning. On a hot day, I like to soak my cleansing pads in water and then leave them in the freezer to chill. Simple but oh so effective and, so long as you have access to a freezer, it's absolutely free.

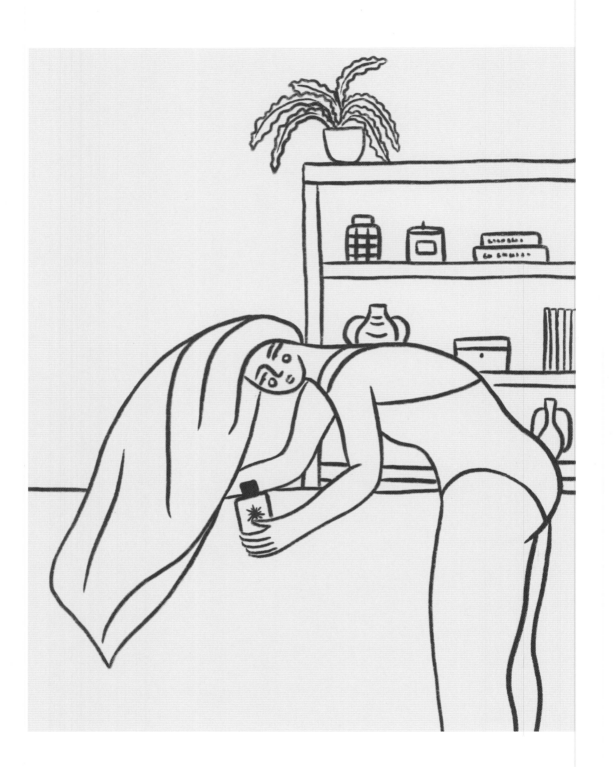

Sunburn and Peeling

Aloe Vera

Nature's own after-sun. The aloe plant is a tropical
succulent with excellent **hydrating** (see p. 54)
and calming properties. If you're lucky enough
to be holidaying in the Caribbean and happen to
have an aloe vera plant in the garden, try cracking
open one of its leaves and smearing the gelatinous
contents over your sunburn or insect bites. It smells
awful and is very sticky, but will instantly soothe
and reduce redness. Failing that, look for an after-
sun lotion that contains aloe vera extract (not simply
a synthetic aloe fragrance).

Lavender

See p. 108 for information on lavender essential oil,
but I've also included lavender here because it's a
little-known fact that it's a brilliant soothing treatment
for mild burns. I rub a little into my fingertips any time
I accidentally nip them with my curling tongs.

Peeling

The beauty editor equivalent to the walk of shame;
evidence that you've been neglecting skin's
hydration levels and **SPF** application (see p. 94).
Peeling usually happens after your skin has switched
climates or environments, but it can also be a sign
that the skin's natural barrier (the stratum corneum)
has been compromised and needs some TLC. If this
is the case, resist the urge to scrub the hell out of it
and instead show it some love with a non-fragrance
barrier **repair cream** (see p. 119) or, if you know that
essential oils (see p. 83) don't irritate your skin,
a natural rose cream such as Dr Hauschka's.

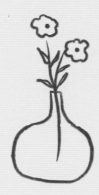

Your SPF Brief

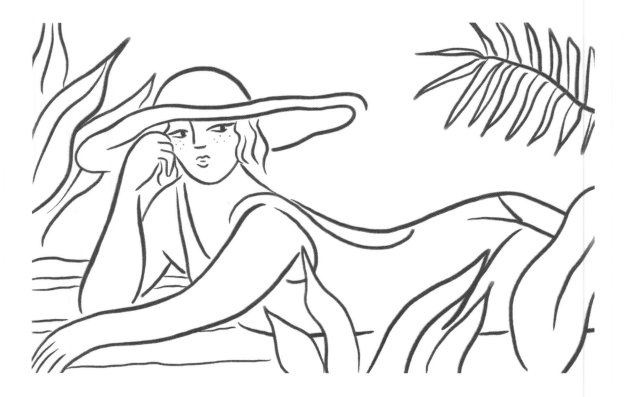

1.

First, cleanse your face and roll with your usual skincare regime.

2.

Next, choose your SPF: physical or chemical, embedded in your skincare or makeup, or as an extra layer in a lotion or mist. I prefer to keep my SPF as a separate product/layer because then I'm fully in control of the amount I apply and when I apply it, and I won't dilute its efficiency by mixing it with moisturizer. A mist is brilliant for this, as you can finish your regular skincare regime, then simply spray over the top. Easy peasy.

3.

Apply the SPF all over your face. This sounds obvious, but if you're using a bronzer or tinted moisturizer with SPF embedded in it, instead of a separate lotion/mist, it needs to cover your whole face – not just your T-zone or cheekbones – in order to be effective.

4.

You don't need to take your makeup off to reapply sunscreen to your face but you may want to touch up after, if you get my gist! There are some clever, desk-friendly SPFs: I love the Sisley Super Stick Solaire, which is easy to use and tops up your colour at the same time, Pixi's Sun Mist SPF30, and Dr Barbara Sturm's Mini Sun Drops.

5.

Reapply throughout the day. The amount you need to reapply depends on both your skin tone (see the Fitzpatrick scale, p. 196) and the factor. On holiday or in direct sunshine you need to be really diligent with this – sun damage is the number one cause of skin ageing. If you don't have more SPF, stay in the shade.

6.

If you're on holiday and swimming, check to see whether your sunscreen is waterproof, otherwise you'll need to reapply once you've dried off.

7.

At the end of the day, take your sunscreen off. You don't need to wear SPF to bed, so thoroughly cleansing or double cleansing your skin at night is important. If your face cream has SPF in it, don't use it as a night cream too.

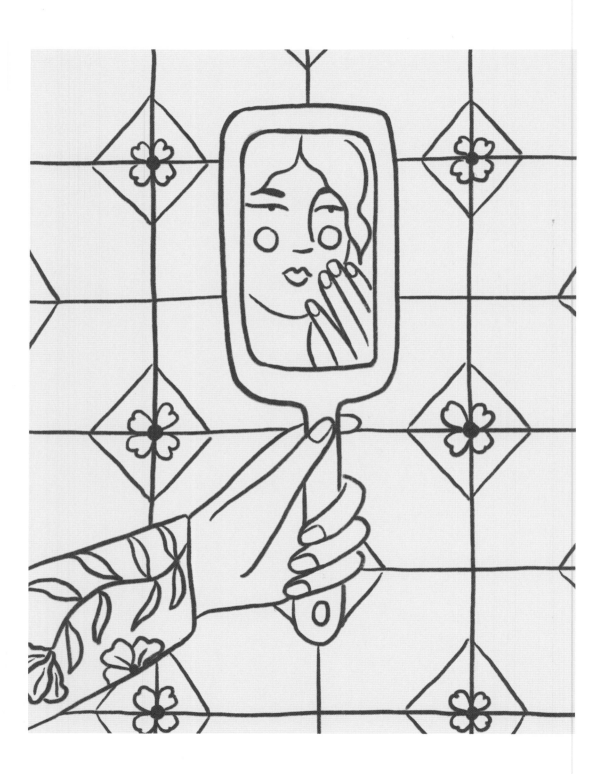

On the Spot

Acne

Acne, an infection of the sebaceous glands, affects nearly 80% of the UK's population, and it can strike at any age; in fact, cases of adult acne in cities such as London are higher than ever before. The most important thing to remember about acne is that no one has to suffer through it. There is always a solution, whether that's topical, treatments-based, or lifestyle- and diet-led. There is always something to be done. While this book lists different ingredients and products that you can try at home to help zap zits (see **drying lotion**, right; **salicylic acid**, p. 129; and **sulphur**, p. 131), you also have the option of going to the dermatologist, who can prescribe anything from a course of **acid peels** (see p. 139) to **antibiotics** (below), **Roaccutane** (p. 129) and **Tretinoin** (p. 149).

Acne Patches

These little patches of skincare-infused plastic or cellulose (like tiny sheet masks) are embedded with spot-busting ingredients. Traditionally they look functional, but model Charli Howard has launched a cute range shaped like flowers and decorated with crystals for her brand Squish.

Antibiotics

Dermatologists sometimes prescribe low doses of antibiotics to help clear up a bout of persistent spots. While this can be a swift and effective solution, given the frightening, impending antibiotics resistance crisis it's best to save them for last-resort situations (if at all). There are plenty of other options to explore, whether natural, holistic or medicinal. **Acupuncture** (p. 133), for example, can be a great holistic alternative, while **manuka honey** (p. 34) and **turmeric** (p. 39) are super natural ones; **salicylic acid** (p. 129) and **Roaccutane** (p. 129) are highly effective hi-tech alternatives.

Bacne

Pimples on your back are really hard to get rid of once you've got them. Try booking in for a back facial or a hammam scrub to deep-clean and unblock pores.

Drying Lotion

These peptobismol pink solutions are brilliant at shrinking spots overnight. My advice? Keep one in every bathroom and every washbag you own; I recommend Kate Somerville EradiKate or Mario Badescu Drying Lotion. Most contain a separated mixture of clear liquid and pink or beige gunk (like oil and vinegar in a salad dressing). Instead of shaking them together, dip a Q-tip into the bottle down through each layer and then dab over and around your blemish, leaving it to work its magic overnight. LIFESAVING.

Inflammation

Nine-tenths of what makes a spot so awkwardly visible is a result of swelling. Inflammation and redness unfortunately make a mountain out of what is otherwise a molehill. But the good news is that if you can quickly reduce that inflammation (see, for example, **sulphur**, p. 131, and **zinc oxide**, p. 95), then you can drastically shrink the size of the spot.

Salicylic acid

"Salicylic acid is a key ingredient for daily unclogging of pores. I often include it in my face and bodycare regime.

The Paula's Choice 2% BHA Liquid Exfoliant is my go-to for bulldozing dry, textured skin around the nose and forehead. I add a few drops to a cotton pad and sweep it all over for a complexion wake-me-up.

For the body, I use CeraVe's Renewing SA Cleanser to break down any dead, flaky skin."

Sarah Jossel, Beauty Director, *Sunday Times Style*
#thebeautyboss

Roaccutane

This **vitamin A** (see p. 112) derivative is taken orally and prescribed by a doctor or dermatologist to treat severe **acne** (see p. 127). So how does it work? Roaccutane shrinks the size of the oil glands and reduces the amount of oil produced by the gland by about 80%. We know it works but it comes with a price; the side effects, depending on the dosage and the skin type, can be vicious. I've seen friends and family members on low doses with painful sores the size of walnuts over their legs and arms, and with peeling, inflamed knuckles. Your acne may get worse before it gets better, too. There are even cases, albeit rare, where Roaccutane can affect the user's mental health, increasing the risk of mood swings and depression. A high price to pay for an acne cure…

Salicylic Acid

Forget witch hazel: this resurfacing whizz-kid ingredient should be a staple in any anti-acne skincare regime. I like to apply a small amount of a cream that contains it – such as Mario Badescu Anti-Acne Serum – to a specific breakout, and I often use it after a flight.

Saline

Have you ever noticed how a week at the beach can clear up bad skin? The salt water in the ocean (along with the burst of sunshine, plenty of rest, and exfoliation of the sand) can help dry out skin and deep-clean pores. Beauty editors like to call it "Vitamin Sea". So will a DIY cleanse with salt water mixed up at home have the same effect? It's certainly one of my favourite basic beauty tricks, and I swear it dries out my skin nicely when it's feeling super oily … BUT I wouldn't recommend it every day since acne-prone skin needs **hydrating** ingredients (see p. 54) to correct sebum imbalance.

★

Squeezing

No one has completed any scientific studies to prove that squeezing your spots is addictive, but I think we can safely assume it is. Seeing as it's unlikely the human race will stop squeezing pimples any time soon, here are a few pointers:

ALWAYS wash your hands and thoroughly clean your skin before and after.

**

Do not squeeze or pick if you can see the spot is in any way red or infected.

**

Try not to squeeze, press or pinch directly into the spot. Instead, apply gentle pressure either side, using a tissue between your fingers and your skin.

Toothpaste

"Toothpastes in the past have contained hydrogen peroxide, which can be an irritant when applied to skin, and triclosan, which is an antibacterial agent that would also have helped to clear up spots.

However, both these agents are completely out of favour due to their side effects, and there are some very good reasons why companies should not use them, including the fact that triclosan has been implicated in bowel cancer whilst hydrogen peroxide, if ingested, can be damaging to the liver.

Many toothpastes also contain sodium lauryl sulphate, which can be an irritant when applied to the skin."

Shabir Daya, Co-founder of Victoria Health

Sulphur

A brilliant bacteria-busting ingredient. Luckily, most **clay** (see p. 133) face masks and spot lotions that use it don't smell nearly half as bad as you would imagine, and some are really great at reducing the **inflammation** (see p. 127) around a spot in just one night.

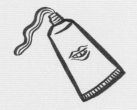

Tea Tree

This is a natural antiseptic and anti-inflammatory, hence it's used in plenty of high-street anti-blemish cleansers and spot treatments. Is it the most effective spot treatment? No, I would always recommend reaching for a **drying lotion** (see p. 127) containing **sulphur** (see above) in zit emergencies, but tea tree is certainly a great natural addition for those following an anti-blemish skincare routine or trying to cut down the synthetics on their bathroom shelf. If you're suffering with **bacne** (see p. 127) or blocked pores on your chest, adding a couple of drops to a warm bath won't do any harm and may even clear up your problem spots.

Toothpaste

The oldest trick in the beauty book, and one that isn't totally an old wives' tale. There are some ingredients in some toothpastes that will dry out a spot: baking soda, menthol and **triclosan** (p. 91) are three examples. However, that doesn't mean that dotting it over your skin at night is going to be more beneficial than a custom-made spot treatment. Plus toothpaste contains all sorts of other ingredients that aren't designed to be applied to your skin. Go figure.

Zinc Oxide

See p. 95 for zinc oxide as a mineral sunscreen, but NB it can also reduce the **inflammation** (see p. 127) and redness that surround a spot.

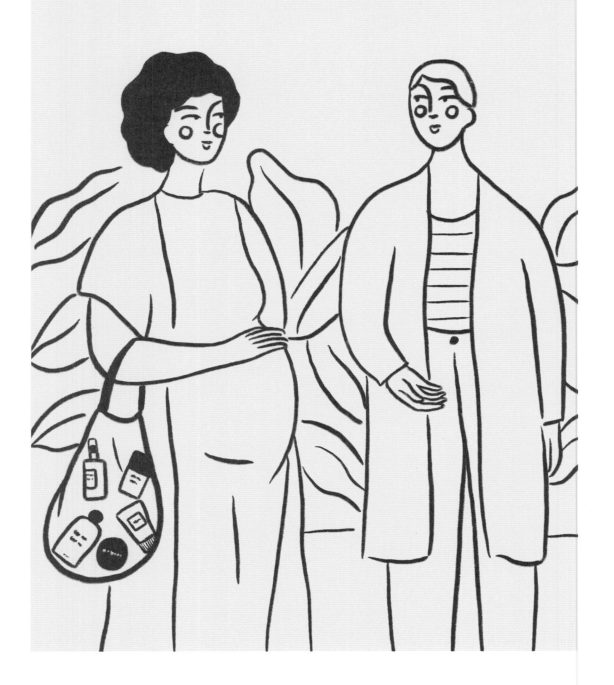

Hormonal Skin

Acupuncture

If your hormones are out of whack, then no amount of sebum-regulating ingredients are going to stop your spots from reappearing time and again. You have to treat the root of the problem, and acupuncture can be a really efficient and relaxing (so long as you're not afraid of needles) therapy for doing so. Instead of inserting needles into the skin around the problem area, the acupuncturist will choose points all over the body that rebalance your endocrine (hormone) system and, by proxy, should clear up your skin.

Clay

A great, gentle oil absorber of excess sebum (which can be a result of hormones, but also stress, environment and diet), clay has been used for centuries, if not millennia, in skincare, and you can find it on the market in lots of different varieties. Some of my favourites for their gentle detoxing effects are **kaolin clay** (see p. 76) and French green clay.

"Clay is one of Mother Nature's wonder ingredients. Straight out of the earth in varying types and colours, nothing beats using clay in a formulation for drawing out impurities and detoxifying the skin. It's one of the most natural ingredients out there that we can use, and in my opinion it gives one of the best results."

Haley Bloom Fitzpatrick, New Product Developer

Cystic Acne

That deep, underground **acne** (see also p. 127) that appears to have no head and that throbs with pain and pressure. It seems to get worse as you get older... Sorry. These spots are different from regular whiteheads and blackheads, as the infection goes deep within your skin, forming a cyst that fills with pus.

Beauty Editor Tip
—
"Whatever you do, don't try to pop or squeeze cystic acne. It won't budge, and it will just make it worse. Instead, hold an ice cube over it. This will constrict the blood vessels feeding the cyst and decrease its appearance rapidly."

Melasma

For this often hormone-related form of hyperpigmentation, it would be wise to look to a fragrance-free, hypoallergenic brand such as La Roche Posay. It may also be worth visiting your GP or dermatologist.

Oestrogen

The baby-making hormone. As with all hormones, when oestrogen levels in your body change this will have a knock-on effect on the way skin behaves — namely, it will start producing a lot more sebum. If you don't manage this with skincare (gentle resurfacing and decongesting), the result is often hormonal breakouts. Fluctuations can occur for all kinds of reasons — time of the month, lifestyle changes, stress and pregnancy.

Pregnancy Skin

A Brazilian social media editor friend of mine once told me that in Brazil the saying goes that having a boy makes you more beautiful, and having a girl sucks the beauty from you! Having just had my first baby, I could bore you to tears with the ups and downs and swings and roundabouts of antenatal skin. But every pregnancy is different, so here's a general list of product changes that you might want to make as you move through each trimester.

◇ In the first trimester, ditch your products with **essential oils** (p. 83) or strong synthetic **fragrance** (p. 30) — especially lemongrass essential oil, as this can promote menstruation. Roll with any bad skin or spots, as they will almost certainly get better.

◇ In the second trimester, your skin might perk up a bit and breakouts calm down, so focus on maximizing your pregno-glow — from all the extra blood that's pumping through you and from all that water you're drinking because, yes, you'll be parched from rising levels of progesterone. Try rosemary, argan and rosehip oils (the De Mamiel Pregnancy Facial Oil is brilliant). I also added a spoonful of coconut oil to my bath each night and didn't get a single stretch mark (though genetics may have played a part, as well as lots of massage and yoga).

◇ In the third trimester, you'll be exhausted and everything will be an effort; even lying on your back for a facial will seem impossible. My advice: stick to multitasking ingredients that make your

life easier, such as cleansing balms that remove your makeup, or **micellar waters** (see p. 41). Infuse your skin with as many moisturizing ingredients as you can because the weeks post-birth will rinse your natural resources, leaving you dehydrated. It's up to you whether you want to use exclusively natural products, but my personal advice is to use products that will help manage the extra sebum you're producing and clean out your pores in a gentle way. I recommend quitting your **retinol** products (see p. 112) throughout pregnancy, since skin may be more sensitive.

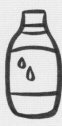

5. SOS

Hormonal Skin

"It's long been known that our hormones affect the condition of our skin, yet little innovation has ever been devoted to helping women control the fluctuations that occur throughout their hormonal cycle.

Now beauty brands are taking inspiration from the wellness industry and creating products aligned with natural human cycles and chronobiology. They are launching platforms that make it easier to understand the menstrual cycle and helping women harness biological and meteorological rhythms, from unique sleep solutions to hormone-targeted supplements.

The Moody website, for example, is designed to help women understand their biology better and enable them to 'live their best life'. In a similar vein, US brand Knours aims to demystify women's changing beauty needs by tracking the user's monthly cycle and collating this with medical insights.

Pushing the time-body connection further, brands are now breaking down beauty routines day by day, or even hour by hour, encouraging ritualized applications and offering purpose-led solutions."

Victoria Buchanan, Senior Futures Analyst at The Future Laboratory and Co-founder of The Beauty Conversation

6

At the Derm

Your Guide to Skincare Procedures

Pots of face cream will promise you the world, but the reality is there is only so much they can do. You can hand over as much money as you like but the absolute most they can achieve, whether they contain pure gold, snake venom or fairy dust, is to gradually reduce the appearance of skin imperfections over time. For a more instant or hard-hitting solution, you might want to visit a facialist or a dermatologist who can perform advanced skin treatments and non-surgical cosmetic enhancements, and, in the case of the dermatologist, prescribe more medicinal solutions. However, while the demand for non-surgical treatments has risen steadily, this really is an area in which you need to do your research. A whole spectrum of people are qualified to perform these treatments, and will sell them to you for an even larger spectrum of prices. As a general rule, beware discounted offers or group bookings; and always get a consultation first. Here is my A–Z of things you need to know.

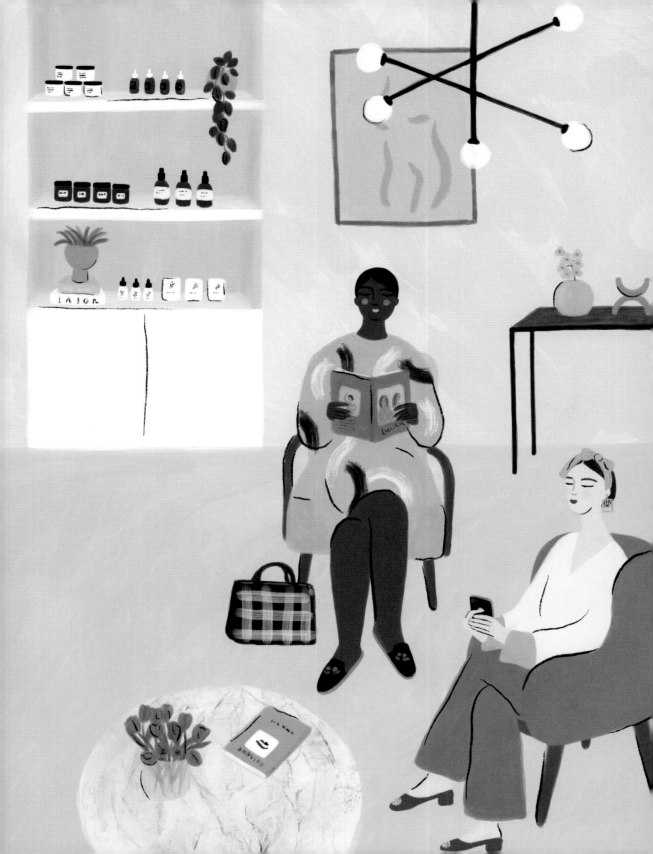

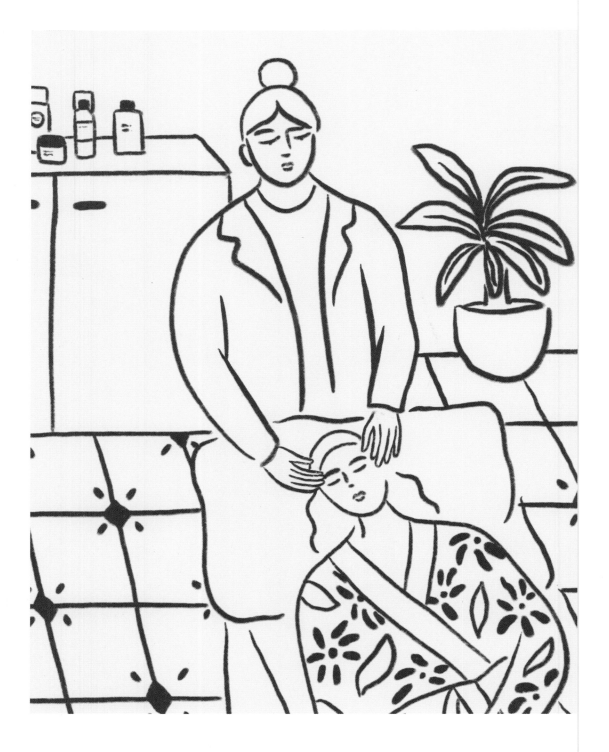

Treatments

3D Face Mapping

This is a really fun and genuinely insightful element to add into your **consultation** (see p. 159). A 3D scanner is used to map out a 360° image of your face. The software can be used to see what you would look like with two left or two right sides in order to better spot asymmetry. Spooky but fun.

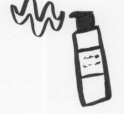

Acid Peels

Otherwise known as chemical peels. An application of a medical-grade acid to the skin kick-starts or speeds up the process of **cell renewal** (see p. 103). At the dermatologist, these acids are likely to be in a much higher concentration than you would get on the high street and may leave you with a red face. The treatment won't hurt, but it will tingle or prickle. The facialist or dermatologist might tap your skin with their fingers to distract you from any discomfort. Some acid peels won't be advisable for darker skin tones or sensitive skin types: always do your research.

Acupuncture Facials

A traditional facial that incorporates acupuncture localized over the face. The idea is to increase the blood flow (by piercing or damaging the skin, the body's natural response is to send a flood of healing white blood cells to the area) and kick-start all sorts of good things, like **collagen** synthesis (see p. 30) and **cell renewal** (see p. 103) and repair. Some acupuncturists won't give facials, since they're purely aesthetic, and prefer to address skin problems indirectly through treating other organs and systems in the body, such as your endocrine or digestive systems.

★ (\$)

Anti–Blue Light

The glare of light that is emitted from digital screens is also emitted from the sun, but obviously an iPhone is generally in much closer proximity to your face. There is mounting evidence to suggest that this frequency of light can affect both brain function and the skin adversely. In skin, blue light can induce oxidative stress, which means it creates free-radical damage and promotes premature ageing and the formation of wrinkles. This light can penetrate deep into the skin, and it also affects our levels of melatonin, which is the sleep hormone, which means it can disrupt our circadian rhythm, too, and the way that skin cells repair themselves overnight.

Anti–Cellulite

Contrary to popular belief, cellulite is not a type of fat. You won't get it from eating too much chocolate, and it doesn't pile on when you miss a gym session. Cellulite is actually the dimpled texture that is created when the layers of **collagen** fibres (see p. 30) in your skin start to slacken and the underlying fat cells push up from underneath. There are plenty of factors that can weaken your collagen fibres (hormones, ageing, lack of exercise, sudden weight gain) but also plenty of factors that can reduce the resulting cellulite, including massage, cryotherapy, laser treatments and exercise.

CoolSculpting

This fat-freezing procedure uses a cooling device to non-surgically remove the fat cells from certain areas of the body, such as stomach, love handles, bra rolls, double chin, and the scientifically termed "bingo wings". CoolSculpting is FDA-approved and works by destroying fat cells with -7°C cooling. The body then gradually flushes out the dead fat cells and the brand claims you can lose up to inches, plus the results are relatively quick. It can be quite harsh on the skin, and some people report that it's quite a painful treatment, but, as we know, tolerable pain varies considerably from person to person. A couple of words of warning about this popular treatment: 1) Do not have it the week before a holiday. I have heard of cases where women have experienced pigmentation issues with immediate sun exposure. 2) I have met beauty editors who have been left with small indents or dimples from the treatment. Just saying...

Crystal Facials

Pretty much what it says on the tin. This is a facial in which crystals are placed around and on your body, and crystal face-massaging tools might be used as well. Does it work? That totally depends on how open-minded you are. I certainly find them very peaceful.

Dermabrasion

This skin-resurfacing procedure uses a motorized tool to buff away the outer layers of the skin. No mean treatment, it requires a local anaesthetic to numb the sensation and will leave your skin red and sensitive for weeks. This is definitely one for fair skin types only, as it may cause skin discoloration on darker skin tones. So who would do it, and why? By removing the top layers of skin, you end up revealing skin underneath that is younger-looking, with a decreased appearance of wrinkles, **sun spots** (see p. 95) and facial scarring. Depending on the area of skin being treated, it can be very expensive, however – particularly when you bear in mind that the effects won't last forever.

Dermarollers

A hand-held facial tool that is covered in needles, a dermaroller is rolled over the face in order to create small punctures in the skin. It sounds like an instrument of torture, but in fact it's a clever way of maximizing the effect of topical skincare, and because the punctures are far enough apart to allow for a wound-healing response to occur, essentially you grow new skin. You can now buy at-home **microneedling** kits (see p. 146). For obvious reasons, the needles won't be as long or as effective as professional tools (if you can't trust yourself not to squeeze a spot or attack your cuticles with clippers, then you definitely shouldn't be left alone with a professional-grade dermaroller!), so the penetration of the skin won't be as great and less **collagen** (see p. 30) will be produced. However, using a microneedling tool at home *will* help increase the absorption of your **active** skincare (see p. 49), especially serums that also promote collagen synthesis, as the channels it creates act like funnels to suck down the goodness deeper into the dermis. The advantage of at-home rolling is the price: you can pick up a dermaroller for well under £40 ($50), whereas a pro treatment will set you back more like upwards of £250 ($300). So when not to roll? Do not roll over eczema, broken skin, warts or **cystic acne** (see p. 133). And if you're a **retinol** user (see p. 112), try to come off it at least four days before you roll.

"I love a dermaroller, and I also show clients how to use them at home. The one that I really like is the GloPRO, which has an LED light as well for healing and calming. I use one a couple of times a week when I put on my actives. If you're dermarolling at home, it's best to do it early evening because if there's any redness then obviously you're sleeping through it and it goes down by morning."

Nichola Joss, Facialist

Dermasanding

Unlike **dermarolling** (see opposite), dermasanding is a surgical procedure. Definitely do not try this at home. An abrasive material is used to scrape off the surface layers of skin (it's also known as "skin buffing") in order to lessen the appearance of **acne** scarring (see p. 127), pigmentation and other skin texture issues. You skin may take up to two weeks to heal from the treatment. Facialists are often divided as to whether dermasanding for purely cosmetic reasons is a good idea. Those with a more holistic approach to skin will tell you it's too aggressive, and those with a penchant for heavy-duty, functional machinery will say it's not. It's expensive, too – around £1,000 ($1,300) for a full face.
💰 💰

"Dermasanding is a very niche treatment. I personally prefer less abrasive and 'cleaner' techniques such as dermaplaning (using a scalpel blade) to reduce pigmentation, as there's less risk

of irritation and post-inflammatory pigmentation, particularly in darker skin types, where this can be an issue."

Dr David Jack, Cosmetic Surgeon and Skincare Expert

Eartox

It's not my intention to give you a complex, but some people do apply treatments to their earlobes. Injecting with either **Botox** (see p. 153) or **fillers** (see p. 155) using **hyaluronic acid** (see p. 33) is supposed to plump fine lines and add volume to either drooping or wrinkled earlobes. A numbing cream would be applied to the area first, and it's popular with people who have a penchant for heavy earrings.
💰 💰

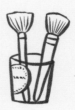

Facials

"When I have the time, I always try to have regular facials with an amazing facialist. If I'm in London I visit Anna Marie Olsen or Debbie Thomas's skin clinic, or when I'm travelling I'll visit Georgia Louise in New York for an amazing, rejuvenating facial. I've worked with Georgia at the incredible Victoria's Secret show as she prepped the gorgeous Angels' skin!"

Charlotte Tilbury, Makeup Artist and Brand Founder

Facials

These are treatments carried out by a facialist, beauty therapist or dermatologist, who cosmetically treat the skin on the face, neck and chest. Facials generally follow the basic road map of **double cleansing** (see p. 45), masking, peeling, massaging and moisturizing.

★ 💰 – 💰 💰

Fat Freezing

These treatments use extreme cold (about -7°C) to kill fat cells. We know that fat cells are very, very tricky. The number of your fat cells is set at adolescence, and when you put on weight your individual fat cells grow in size rather than multiplying. The same goes for when you lose weight: the fat cells decrease in size rather than number. So the only proven way to stop you putting that weight back on is to kill or remove the fat cell – and freezing (as well as heating) is one way to do this. Certain fat-freezing methods such as **CoolSculpting** (see p. 140) can be quite harsh on the skin.

💰 💰

Beauty Editor Tip
—
"Although fat freezing is backed by science, for some people taking a cold shower in the morning, using a body brush and then taking a walk around the garden is going to be far more beneficial (and cost-effective!). If you're trying these treatments because you'd rather pay money than fix an unhealthy lifestyle, then you need to do some re-evaluating."

Fat Lasering

A high-intensity laser is used to heat up the skin to around 45°C, damaging the fat cells in the targeted area, which studies have shown can then be detoxed from the body by white blood cells over the following weeks. Most treatments don't hurt because they use a cooling device on the surface of the skin while the heating goes on beneath the dermis. The best feel quite pleasant – a little like a hot stone massage.

💰 💰 💰

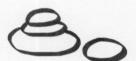

Fractional Radio Frequency Laser

This is one of the many lasers that can be wielded by facialists (not just dermatologists) to reduce the appearance of pigmentation, scarring and fine lines. It uses tiny pins to create channels in the skin to deliver radio frequency into the dermal layers. This then reaches the **collagen** layers (see p. 30) to stimulate and rejuvenate the skin. The idea is that, by damaging the skin, it then has to heal, repair and create new collagen, leaving it healthy and significantly fresher, younger and tighter. This particular laser is safe for use on all skin types and tones.

💰 💰

Fraxel Laser

This brand-named laser should be used with caution on darker skin types, since it can burn the skin or cause hyper/hypo pigmentation.

⊗ 💰 💰

Gala Glow Facial

Performed by one of London's most exciting young derms, Dr Marwa Ali, the Gala Glow facial uses Hifu (high intensity focused ultrasound) and Vitamin C in combination. So good, I'm told you only need to have it once or twice a year.

Infrared (IR)

A certain wavelength of light that is emitted by the sun, infrared can also be produced at a safe level by mechanical cosmetic devices in order to firm up skin texture on the face and body (note it is a skin-firming treatment, not a fat-killing treatment), to stimulate sluggish hair follicles, and to improve stretch marks. You'll also find infrared lamps in yoga studios to increase flexibility via heat, without the drying, dehydrating effect that regular blow heaters have on the skin and body. It's an invigorating sort of heat, similar to the feeling of the sun on your skin in winter, which is why infrared lamps are popular with people who suffer from Seasonal Affective Disorder. Infrared light has been proven to stimulate fibroblasts in the skin to produce more **collagen** (see p. 30) and **elastin** (see p. 111) perfectly safely, but the long-term safety – as with so many things in the world of aesthetics – hasn't yet been properly studied. That for me is a red flag.

Jade Rollers

These massage tools are often double-ended and made from a precious stone or crystal such as jade, rose quartz or tourmaline. They have been used in Chinese skincare regimes (to massage serums and oils into the skin) for hundreds, if not thousands, of years. The immediate effect is a boost in circulation and skin vitality, and increased lymphatic drainage. You might even come across a facial where two rollers are used in tandem, which requires impressive dexterity from the therapist. So are the benefits increased by the mere fact that the tool might be made of crystal? Well, that depends on your take on the healing properties of crystals. There's certainly no harm in using one, and at the very least the stone will feel cool and soothing on your skin.

Kybella

A fat-dissolving injection that has been FDA-approved only for use under the chin, this is deployed off-label by dermatologists on other areas of the body. It uses a naturally occurring molecule that assists in the destruction and absorption of fat cells and takes about two shots to work.

LED Light Facials

A glorious, non-scary, **non-invasive** (see p. 160) way to get your glow back, and a brilliant way to manage breakouts. LED facials have been enormously popular in Australia and LA for ages, but it's only recently that cities like London and New York have cottoned on to the power of a weekly dose of light therapy (see also **white light facials**, p. 150). Your therapist will cover your eyes with protective glasses, and then shine an LED lamp over your skin. The feeling of bright warmth is also wonderfully mood-boosting – a little holiday in a facial – and you'll come out of this treatment feeling as buoyant and radiant as you look.

★

"LED facials, in or out of clinic, can be nice treatments, and there can be positive effects treating acne, pigmentation and other skin issues, but in reality very regular treatments are required to really see significant, sustainable changes."

Dr David Jack, Cosmetic Surgeon and Skin Expert

Lip Blushing

This treatment adds semi-permanent pigment to the lips to make them look fuller – the latest alternative to lip filler, apparently!

Mesotherapy

This consists of lots of tiny little injections all over the face to pepper the surface of the skin with a cocktail of vitamins, minerals and naturally occurring moisturizing factors such as **hyaluronic acid** (see p. 33). The aim is to plump up the skin over the entire face, rather than in just localized areas, and the end result is much less drastic than **Botox** (see p. 153). You'll look like you've had a month of really great sleep, plus your face still moves freely. It can, however, be combined with Botox to help soften deep wrinkles.

Microblading

If you haven't seen the *Vogue* video featuring actress and activist Lena Dunham getting her eyebrows microbladed, then I recommend you do so. Microblading (or nanoblading) is essentially when a therapist wielding a hand-held tool places pigment under the skin, in the shape of individual eyebrow strokes. It's not the same as tattooing, but it does help to boost the apparent volume of your brows, making them look fuller and shapelier; friends have raved about the transformative effect it has on their face. Though people's pain thresholds do vary, it reportedly isn't as painful as tattooing either: the skin underneath your brow is numbed while the shape of the brow is first sketched on, and most say the microblading feels similar to having the point of a compass scratched gently over the skin.

A word of warning: the first week is always a bit of a shock, as your eyebrows will look quite stark and potentially darker than you would like. As the colour starts to fade, though, they come into their own and look more realistic. Also worth noting is that if you have dark skin and use an **anti-pigmentation** cream (see p. 97), you may be fading the pigment a little quicker, so try to avoid the brow area.

Microchanneling

Another name for **microneedling** (see p. 146).

Microdermabrasion

The little sister of **dermabrasion** (see p. 140), microdermabrasion is non-surgical (meaning that non-medical **facialists** can offer it on their menus; see p. 159). It uses a tool to remove only the dead layers of surface skin without damaging the living layers.

Microneedling

This is when a **dermaroller** (see p. 140) is used as part of a facial treatment to improve the texture of your skin.

Oxygen Facials

A standard facial during which oxygen is blasted at your skin. The immediate results are a bright, vitalized glow and increased plumpness. I love them before an event for instant "wow" factor. However, most oxygen facials are very expensive, given that the benefits rarely last that long, and unless you're having one a week you're unlikely to get enough prolonged payback for your cash. In fact, you may see similar results from an outdoor workout, and at least you'll have burned some calories at the same time. I think we often forget the power of breath and oxygenating our organs (of which our skin is one). Having a facial that encourages you to breathe as part of the process, or doing a breath meditation class, is going to oxygenate your skin more efficiently than most creams can. You can also find facials that are carried out in oxygenated rooms, which obviously will be beneficial to both the way you look and feel.

Peel Bars

These drop-in-style facial bars, instead of mixing up margaritas for their customers, deliver a menu of **acid peels** (see p. 139). Now commonplace in cities such as London, New York and LA, where fast-paced, accessible beauty is the norm, these bars are usually manned by a dermatologist who specializes in peels, but legally it could just be an aesthetician, so do your research.

Plastic Surgery

The fact that plastic surgery is called "plastic" interestingly has nothing to do with the implants used being made from plastic. The word is actually derived from the Ancient Greek "plastikos", meaning to shape or mould. So what are implants actually made from? Synthetic implants (for breast and bum) can be made from silicone that contains either a silicone gel or a saline solution, whereas autologous implants are when a person's tissue is extracted from their body, processed and then re-injected into a different part of the body that needs reshaping.

Radiofrequency

This is sold as the skin-tightening treatment for those who want an alternative to going under the knife. It's completely **non-invasive** (see p. 160) and works by using a machine to heat the skin to 38–40°C in order to create more **collagen** (see p. 30), which lifts and firms the skin. It works everywhere, from your butt to your **marionette lines** (see p. 156). You can even get the skin around your nether regions treated – a popular one post-partum. The major benefits are that it's quick (your whole face will take about half an hour), there's no **downtime** (see p. 159), and the lower frequencies can get deeper into the skin than lasers to improve skin texture. The downside? It's about £200 ($250) for half an hour and you're going to want to book in for a course of six or so to get the best results.

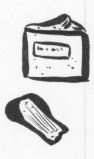

Oxygen Facials

"The term 'oxygen facial' is a confusing
one, as most facials are actually more
about delivering high-concentration vitamins
into the skin on an oxygen-carrier system,
rather than oxygen itself. Without a doubt,
these ingredients are good for the skin,
but in oxygen facials that are done once
every couple of months for ten minutes
it's unlikely there will be significant,
sustained cellular changes. Any benefit
is more likely to come from vitamins used
in addition."

Dr David Jack, Cosmetic Surgeon and Skin Expert

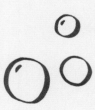

Touch therapy

"On a holistic, self-love level, facial massage removes negativity from the day which can be embedded in your muscle tissue. It's like a meditative process, like a physical meditation. You can also incorporate breath work into it - breathing in deeply, breathing out, as you're massaging, to help dispel everything. That slow massage and breathing also gets your body ready for sleep, and when your body is ready for sleep it can address your skin, so your skin cell renewal process will actually activate quicker and will work better for you."

Nichola Joss, Facialist

Retinoic Acid (Tretinoin)

A form of **vitamin A** (see p. 112) that's often prescribed by dermatologists for treatment of severe **acne** (see p. 127). It works by exfoliating dead skin cells and promoting the growth of new, healthier cells. It's a popular ingredient in anti-wrinkle creams, too, but the stuff you get from the dermatologist is likely to be much more concentrated. Any ethnicity can use it, but if you have darker skin and the retinoic acid happens to cause a reaction or irritate the skin then it can sometimes result in hyperpigmentation.

Self-dissolving Microneedle Masks

Quite new to the market, these **sheet masks** (see p. 76) are covered in tiny, barely perceptible microneedles formed from **active** ingredients (see p. 49) such as **hyaluronic acid** (see p. 33) or bio-needles from the freshwater Spongilla sponge. When the needles touch your skin, they create channels through which the sheet-mask serum can be absorbed, then after some minutes they dissolve and also flow into the channels. Clever.

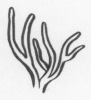

Semi-permanent Makeup

Things have come a long way since the block brows and wobbly lipliners you may have been used to seeing. You can now get organic inks that allow you to change the shape and colour after a year, and that no longer fade away as pink or blue. Semi-permanent freckle tattoos are also now a thing, which I have to admit I would consider, and natural-looking **microblading** (see p. 145) works wonders on many people's facial structure.

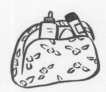

Touch Therapy

This holistic treatment for pain relief and relaxation was developed by a psychic healer in the 1970s. In therapeutic touch (TT), the healer will lay their hands on your body, moving the energy around between the two of you. Whether you believe in the power of healing or not, there's definitely something in it. According to research carried out by the KAO Corporation (the company that owns John Frieda haircare and other global brands), touching of the facial skin by the palm of the hands was found to increase blood flow to areas of the brain's prefrontal cortex, which is known to activate feelings of positivity and pleasure. Interestingly, a second study compared brain activation when different types and textures of cream were applied: the cream that had a rich, moisturizing feel achieved the most significant cerebral blood-flow change.

Ultherapy

Ultrasound's big brother. This non-surgical form of skin firming for both the face and body uses ultrasound waves to boost **collagen** production (see p. 30) in the skin. It also uses regular ultrasound imaging to allow the skin therapist to see the layers of tissue being treated. It's not cheap: we're talking upwards of £750 ($1,000) for one area, and a standard Ultherapy face "lift" will take around an hour.

💰💰💰

Ultrasound Facials

Ultrasound waves have been used in facials for decades to jump-start **collagen** production (see p. 30) and help "push" products deeper into the skin. You can even buy hand-held ultrasound facial massagers for at-home use: the Foreo LED Thermo Activated Smart Mask Device is brilliant and looks cute, too. As a treatment it feels pleasant and relaxing, and it gives you a nice little lift with regular use. But what lots of people don't know is that ultrasound waves also kill bacteria, so it's a great treatment for helping to manage breakouts.

White Light Facials

The white setting of an LED lamp (see also **LED light facials**, p. 144) emits light waves with the longest wavelength, meaning they can travel deeper into the skin. White light facials are now quite common on the high street. They contain zero UV light and are brilliant for energizing sluggish skin.

YAG Laser

Dermatologists and facialists use YAG lasers to break down pigmentation, with the welcome side effect that it kills bacteria in the pores over the course of a series of treatments.

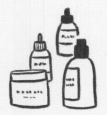

At-Home Laser

"The people behind the nutraceutical
LYMA supplement have recently developed
an at-home, hand-held, pain-free laser,
which reverses the signs of ageing by
stopping cells producing the nitric oxide
that prevents them from absorbing oxygen
and nutrients. It's early days … but
this could change everything."

Annabel Rivkin, Journalist

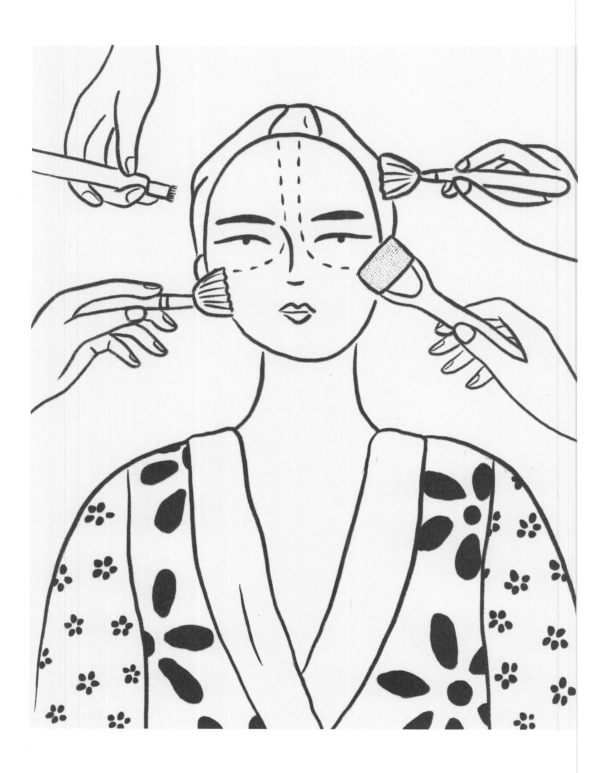

Injectables

Baby Botox

To be clear, this does not mean giving **Botox** (see below) to babies! Baby Botox is a term coined by marketeers to refer to a lower dosage of the toxin. The result, in theory, should be gentler and more subtle, with only partial movement inhibition and not total. Remember: individuals will react differently to Baby Botox (and indeed Botox), and there is no one measure to say how much muscle movement will be inhibited from person to person.

Botox

Botox is the brand name for a biological substance, *Botulinum toxin*, which paralyses human muscle tissue when injected. The Botox brand is owned by Dublin-based pharmaceutical company Allergan, which operates in over one hundred countries and in 2017 registered a net income of over $4 billion (it also owns **Juvederm**; see p. 156). Botox reduces the appearance of fine lines and wrinkles by paralysing the muscles underneath for a limited period of time. It does this by blocking the brain signal from the nerve to the muscle. Essentially, the muscle, which is usually on strict orders from the brain to contract and tighten on demand, will ignore the brain when it tells it to move and, in a bid for freedom, will loosen and relax, causing the wrinkles on top to smooth out.

If you're thinking about having Botox for the first time, you might want to know the following six things, after which you can make up your own mind (unless you're under 18, in which case no Botox for you; though, having said that, in the United States, Botox is FDA-approved for anyone between 18 and 65 but dermatologists and doctors can use it off-label on patients who are younger or older as long as they have the consent of a parent or guardian):

1. Botox does hurt. You'll experience sharp scratches and aching, and likely get tiny bruises or red prick dots around the injection sites. Everyone reacts differently, but you're more than likely to feel an aching, tight, slightly fuggy head feeling for a couple of days, if not more.

2. Botox builds up gradually. You won't notice much difference in the first day or two. Over the following few weeks, day by day, you will wake up to less and less movement in the affected muscles.

3. Once your Botox has taken full effect there's nothing you can do to reverse it until it wears off on its own. This could take 3–6 months depending on the way in which your body processes the toxin. No amount of willing your muscles to move will work.

4. If you naturally emote through your features, you may be surprised by how trapped you feel within your own face. It's a shock for first-time users.

5. Many people who administer Botox (whether that's in a salon, clinic or your best mate's living room) won't tell you the above facts because THEY WANT TO SELL IT TO YOU. Why on earth would they tell you the less glamorous details?!

6. It is important to remember that, although Botox is a brilliant drug that can be used incredibly positively (it has been used to treat illnesses from migraines to strokes, and stops many people grinding their teeth), it is still a potentially deadly poison, and it's a diluted version of this poison that you are injecting into your muscle. It's not the same as an anti-wrinkle cream and it's not a beauty treatment. #Justsaying. But I do use it (sorry mum!).

Botox

"We have to be clear about Botox. It's not an anti-ageing procedure at all. What it's doing is stopping a muscle from moving. By no means does your body completely get rid of it, and by no means is it only that muscle that's affected.

If you're in your twenties and thirties I really don't think you should be doing it, or advocating it to other people in that age group, because we do not have all the scientific evidence as to what it's doing to the rest of our body for our future selves."

Nichola Joss, Facialist

"If you're looking to take your treatment repertoire to the next level, I would recommend starting your search with an accredited listing, e.g. the British Association of Aesthetic Plastic Surgeons website, which has a useful 'Find a Surgeon' directory of trusted, certified surgeons who are all of the highest level of training and qualifications. Just working from London's Harley Street can't guarantee that a practitioner is trustworthy, but such a list can give you a valuable steer."

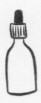

Fillers

Where **Botox** (see p. 153) targets lines on the face by relaxing the muscles underneath them, fillers are injections of fluid that "puff out" these lines, restoring volume to areas of your face that have lost it. If Botox is the steamroller of the injectable world, then fillers are the landscape gardeners. Most commonly, fillers are made from **hyaluronic acid** (see p. 33), a gel-like substance found naturally within your skin with the purpose of binding water to your skin cells. As we age, the hyaluronic acid in our skin stores less water, decreasing the overall volume of the skin. Reinjecting this acid just under the skin can temporarily restore volume and, since the skin recognizes the acid, its tissues won't reject it as a foreign entity. Such filler injections can help restore volume particularly in the nasolabial folds, the **marionette lines** (see p. 156), the tear troughs and the lips, or on the cheekbones and in the lines

on the forehead. Depending on the amount of filler injected, the practitioner will apply a numbing anaesthetic cream to the injection site, but smaller amounts (known to some as "microdosing") tend to only smart as much as vaccination injections. The areas around your nose and mouth tend to be a bit more prickly, due to an abundance of nerve endings. As the filler is injected, you will experience an odd bubbling, popping sensation. The effects of filler can last up to twelve months. You don't need to be a doctor or medical professional to inject it – pretty much anyone can do it, which is scary. I would ALWAYS recommend seeing a medical professional for fillers, and always recommend checking out their work on other people first. Adjusting the surface volume on a face takes a certain amount of artistic skill as well. I have never had fillers and personally it's something I would avoid, as I have seen too many people's faces change fractionally for the worse.

⊗ 💰 💰

Frown Lines

These are the vertical lines that can form between your eyebrows (where your monobrow would grow!) as you age. In beauty slang, they're also known as "elevens" or "frinkles". They're mostly expression lines, caused by frowning, and can be exaggerated by skin dehydration, sun damage and stress, and they can also just be genetic. It's a clever area to treat with **Botox** (see p. 153), since this can gently soften forehead lines while allowing you to maintain the majority of your eyebrow movement.

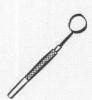

Gums

A gummy smile can be softened using **Botox** (see p. 153), often administered by cosmetic dentists. A smidgen of Botox is injected into the base of each nostril and along the nasolabial lines, which relaxes the top lip and allows it to sit a bit lower over the gums when you smile. It should cost around £150 ($200) and last 3–6 months.

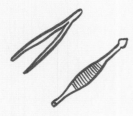

Hyperhidrosis

Botox (see p. 153) can be used to temper excess sweating. Dermatologists in the UK are only licensed to treat the underarm area, though it's not uncommon for facial and hand treatments to slip under the official carpet as a welcome side effect to an aesthetic treatment. For underarms, the injections are placed quite close together and, unfortunately for the patient, as with all Botox, the results wear off after 3–6 months.

Juvederm

This is one of the better-known **hyaluronic acid-based** (see p. 33) brands of dermal **filler** (see p. 155).

Lunchtime Botox

Botox itself (see p. 153) doesn't take long to administer – a couple of minutes at most – but a good practitioner will want to numb your face with a topical anaesthetic cream for 10–20 minutes first, as well as providing you with an in-depth **consultation** (see p. 159). So, yes, in theory you could squeeze all of this into your lunch break, but there certainly wouldn't be time for lunch after. Plus any practitioner in a hurry to inject you shouldn't be trusted. Injecting a toxin into your face should be done with measured consideration and in no rush.

Marionette Lines

Nicknamed "laughter lines", these grooves that bracket the mouth are ironically more likely to make you look grumpy or sad than someone who has spent a lifetime chortling. See **radiofrequency** (p. 146) and **fillers** (p. 155).

Preventative Botox

Many practitioners of **Botox** (see p. 153) will tell you that it can be used as a preventative measure in your early twenties; that by paralysing a facial muscle in young skin you are preventing it from expressing, and therefore stopping wrinkles from forming in the first place. It sounds logical, but could this be a farce to get you to shell out every three to six months for the next seven decades? Well, the answer is yes. There haven't been many studies published on preventative Botox and, as it stands, there is no evidence to say that Botox actually stops wrinkles from forming. Wrinkles may form less aggressively on a young person who has been treated with Botox for years, since studies show that regular usage of Botox encourages muscle atrophy or wastage, but in my opinion if you're injecting Botox before you need it you're simply subjecting your body to years' worth of needless chemicals. It makes no sense to take a drug for something that you don't need.

Restylane

A brand of **hyaluronic acid**-based (see p. 33) facial **filler** (see p. 155), this was one of the first brands to get FDA approval for a lip-specific filler. Restylane uses vegan-friendly hyaluronic acid, meaning it's not animal-derived as some fillers can be.

Tech-neck

A 21st-century problem, staring down at our phones encourages permanent lines, wrinkles and skin sagging. Plus the Zoom boom has meant that we are more aware of said sagging. **Ultherapy** (see p. 150) and **Botox** (see p. 153) are derm solutions, but there are also good lifting creams out there. Or maybe just gaze at your phone less...

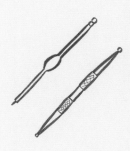

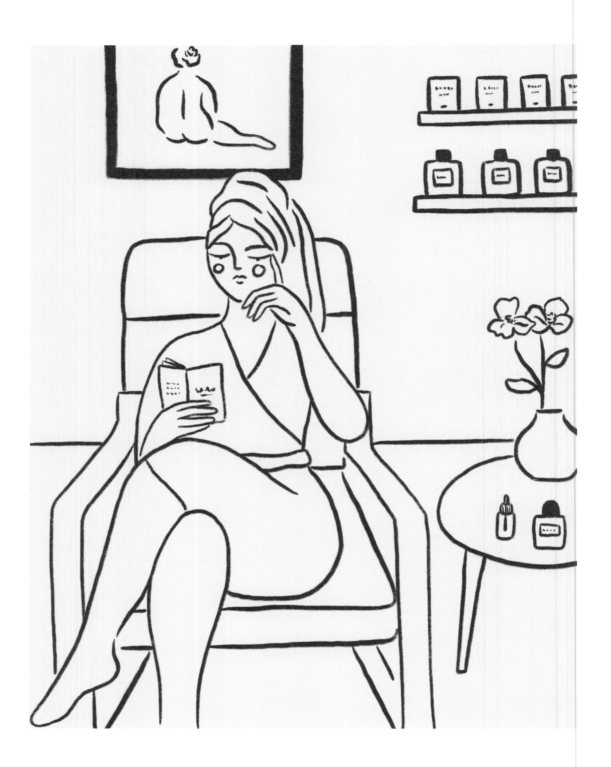

Dermatology Terminology

Clinical Staff

The best tip I could ever pass on as a beauty editor is to closely inspect the faces of the receptionists and assisting nurses when you're in the waiting room of a clinic. The likelihood is that they will have been able to sample the work carried out at the clinic (often at a discount or as a guinea pig) and are therefore a living example of what you can expect the "finish" to look like. This is not law, of course, but in general it's a great rule to live by. Try not to be too obvious in your gawking...

Consultations

Always, always, always go for a consultation first if you're thinking about doing anything dramatic to your face. It's worth every minute.

Dermatologically Tested

This stamp is less a seal of ultimate approval than a mark that the product has been reviewed by at least one dermatologist who decided that it suits all skin types. It is well-meaning in most cases, but is generally a marketing tool to boost consumer confidence in a new product.

Dermatologist-recommended

As above, be wary of this phrase. It simply means that a dermatologist has reviewed the product. Brands can use the phrase regardless of how little the dermatologist rated it.

Downtime

This relates to the amount of time that your face will look or feel different (read: bruised, red, swollen, discoloured, flaky, peeling or tender to touch) after a treatment is performed. I once had a **Fraxel laser** treatment (see p. 143) on a scar on my chin, which left it bright purple for a week. Always ask about downtime, and be prepared to clear your diary.

Facialist

Facialists are skin experts, aestheticians or beauticians who specialize in giving facials. There is no certification required by law to give facials, but many practitioners do have qualifications that are displayed in their salons or clinics. Should you visit a facialist without a qualification? Some of the best are self-taught, or learned their skills as apprentices or assistants to already established facialists. It's often a skill with trade secrets that are handed on. No qualification doesn't always mean no go (unless they are operating heavy machinery or wielding needles).

Invasive

Beauty treatments are dubbed invasive when they physically break the skin. A face lift is invasive; a butt implant is invasive. A Hollywood bikini wax, although it may feel like the most hideously intrusive procedure, is not technically classed as invasive.

Medical Dermatologist

Dermatology is the branch of medicine concerned with the study of the skin, making dermatologists medical doctors who have specialized in skin. Dermatology does, in some cases, cover cosmetic enhancements and care.

Minimally Invasive

This refers to a treatment that is carried out – with or without a dermatologist present – using a tool or ingredient that enters the body through the skin or a cavity but with minimal damage done to the skin's tissues. Injectables such as **Botox** (see p. 153), **fillers** (see p. 155) and **microneedling** (see p. 146) are all classed as minimally invasive.

Non-invasive

Treatments are classed as non-invasive when they don't break the skin. An **LED light facial** (see p. 144) is non-invasive, as is an **acid peel** (see p. 139), but needle-based treatments that puncture the skin, such as **Botox** (see p. 153) and **microneedling** (see p. 146), are not. Also, just because something is labelled "non-invasive", doesn't mean that it won't hurt or can't damage your skin.

Risk-free

Very little in beauty is totally risk-free. Even the mildest ingredients and procedures could have consequences if you have sensitive skin, so always ask your therapist or get a second opinion as to how your unique skin type could react to a treatment.

6. At the Derm

Invasive, Minimally Invasive and Non-invasive

"In plastic surgery we usually use these terms, meaning the following:

'Invasive' refers to medical procedures that 'invade' the body, entering the dermis and subcutaneous tissue through a medical instrument. The vast majority of plastic surgery procedures, such as facelifts, breast augmentation or abdominoplasty, are examples of invasive procedures.

'Minimally invasive' surgery refers to surgical procedures that limit the incision length and the trauma to the body. This can be accomplished with innovative medical technology. In aesthetic surgery it is often done with an endoscope, such as in endoscopic browlifts. Aesthetic procedures, but not surgery, using a syringe are categorized as minimally invasive procedures. These include fillers, neurotoxins, threading, mesotherapy and any other injectables.

'Non-invasive' refers to medical procedures that do not require any incision or injection. Laser, light, LED, Endermologie, temperature treatments, RF, ultrasound and chemical peels qualify as non-invasive and represent a growing repertoire of procedures where technological advances offer effective skin improvement, skin tightening or fat reduction.

The terms do not have a medically accepted level of definition, and for this reason can often be confusing or even misleading. In reality, any procedure requires a degree of invasiveness in order to have a result."

Dr Yannis Alexandrides, Plastic Surgeon
and Co-founder of 111SKIN

The Back of the Bottle

Decoding Cult Products

Just like the B-side of a record, you'll find that some of the best stuff is on the back of the bottle. If you're prepared to get a little geeky, turn your skincare bottle around and there's a lot of useful information to be found on the reverse – information that is often legally there for a reason, and that can help you further understand what the product is going to do for your skin.

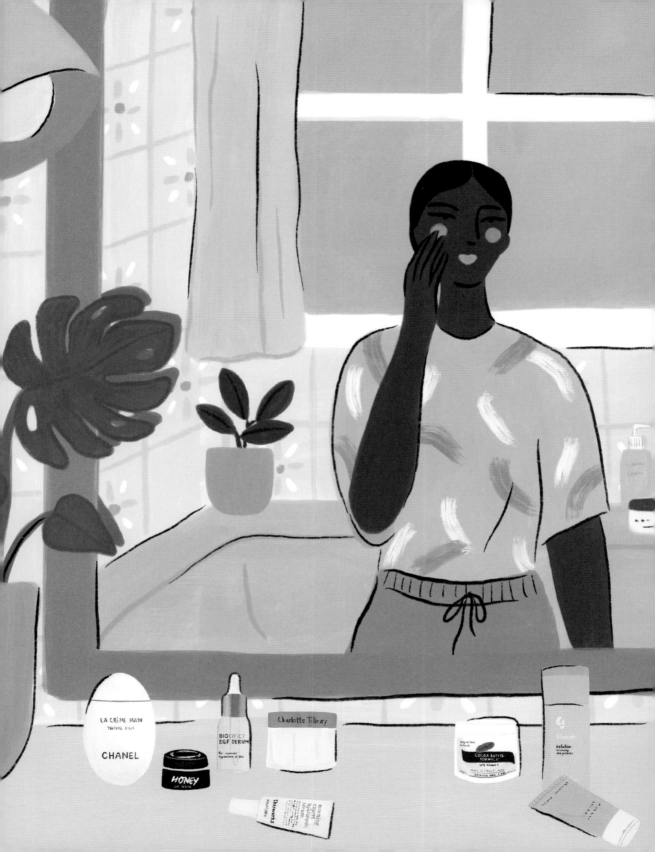

While the information on the front of the label that we have discussed in the Introduction is important, the back of the label is where you can unearth some real truths about the product's contents and cross-reference them with the marketing claims on the front. So what can you find on the reverse of the product?

◆ The INCI listing (the list of ingredients)

◆ The use-by date

◆ The directions for use

◆ The quantity of product contained inside the packaging

◆ The address of the brand's HQ

◆ A series of symbols and logos that indicate the product's status as recyclable, organic, cruelty-free, etc.

For various reasons, however, beauty brands don't make it easy to decipher all this information. For starters, the writing on the reverse of skincare products is often so small you need a magnifying glass to read it. Secondly, a fair amount of it is printed in Latin – not a second language for many people. It's also not always on the back of the bottle: it could be on the side, on the box, or on a folded-up piece of paper inside the packaging. If you're shopping online, this information can be even harder to find, with some global brands not listing their product information at all. That said, shout-out to a few of the game-changing skincare brands helping to demystify the INCI list with radical transparency, such as Typology and The Inkey List. This next section of the book is designed to help you understand what the components are doing there, and how to read them.

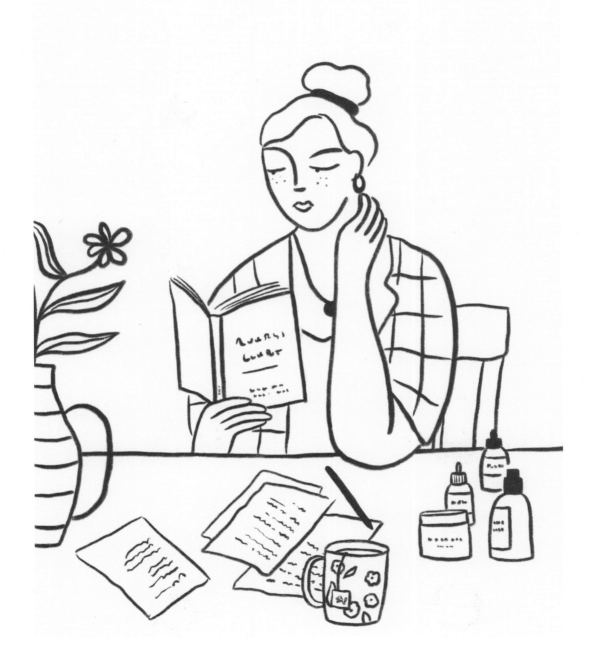

Beauty Iconography

They say pictures speak a thousand words, and in skincare they really do. On the bottle you may have noticed various symbols. Most people are in blissful ignorance of the meaning of these icons, but they're actually extremely useful and make smart shopping a vast amount easier. Once you find out what they mean, you'll kick yourself for not knowing before!

The open pot: The number inside the pot stands for the maximum number of months the product should be used for after opening. So, essentially, it's a use-by date.

The hourglass: If the use-by figure is less than 30 months, the product should carry an hourglass icon, often followed by the use-by date.

The little e: A lowercase "e" is marked on European products at the time of filling to certify the weight of the contents.

Fire, fire! This means the product is flammable. It's probably a hairspray or nail polish remover, or maybe even a deodorant. It doesn't mean it will burn your skin; just don't light a match nearby...

The pointing book: A gentle hint to check further information or instructions within the leaflet provided with the product.

Recycle me: This indicates that the packaging is recyclable. If the symbol is inside a circle and has a percentage inside it, it means that the packaging is itself made from a percentage of recycled materials.

The hugging green arrows: A European symbol that tells you an external company oversees the manufacturer's recycling.

USDA Organic: Valid in the United States, this means the product is at least 95% organic.

ECOCERT: The Ecocert Cosmos certification is used in over 75 countries (including Australia, Brazil, Canada, India and South Korea). It means that at least 95% of the plants a product contains are organic, and over 20% of organic ingredients are present (10% for rinse-off products). The Ecocert Group is one of the largest natural and organic certification bodies in the world.

BIO: The mark of the French organic organization Cosmebio. The word "BIO" stands for "biologique" (the French for organic), and implies that at least 20% of the ingredients of the total product are organic (taking into account water and mineral ingredients which cannot be certified from organic farming), or that at least 95% of the agricultural ingredients in the product are organic.

The Leaping Bunny: The globally recognizable gold standard for cruelty-free consumer products, approved by Cruelty Free International, an audited programme that checks every level of the supply chain to provide the best assurance for consumers.

Cruelty-free bunny: A logo supplied to brands that PETA have certified as "cruelty-free", i.e. they do not allow tests on animals for their products, ingredients or formulations anywhere in the world for any reason.

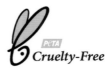

Cruelty-free and vegan bunny: A logo supplied by PETA to brands that do not allow tests on animals for their products, ingredients or formulations anywhere in the world for any reason, and whose products do not contain any animal ingredients.

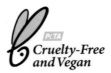

Ban the bin: The wheelie bin with a cross marked over it means, please do not dispose of the product in a regular bin, likely because part of the product contains electronics or batteries.

The INCI List

The International Nomenclature of Cosmetic Ingredients (INCI, often pronounced by industry folks as "inky") is a standardized system of naming cosmetics ingredients. The system was created by the International Nomenclature Committee in 1973 and uses a mixture of scientific names, Latin names, and English "common or usual names". The UK and European listings will always be the same, but the US INCI listings often differ since the US has different legislation and allows some ingredients that are not legal in Europe. Whatever the case, INCI lists are complicated by nature, and even practised beauty editors can scrutinize them and come away relatively none the wiser.

Some important things to know about INCI lists:

♦ The ingredients are listed in weight order, meaning that the ingredient with the highest concentration is always listed first, and then the list reads in descending order of weight from there. This is why for many products you'll notice that aqua (the Latin word for water, the most ubiquitous of all skincare ingredients) is often first up on the list. Normally, the first two—six ingredients are the big ones, while the rest are just included in very small quantities.

♦ There are some ingredients that legally don't need to be included in the INCI list. Also any substance that makes up less than 1% of the weight can be listed at the end in any order. In addition, fragrances don't need to be listed in full, because most synthetic fragrances are made up of a hundred-odd scents, so to list them would require a lot more packaging space and therefore they're all bundled together under the umbrella word "fragrance" or "parfum".

♦ Colorants are generally listed together at the very end of the INCI list. In the EU, they are listed as a series of five-digit codes; in the US, they are listed as a colour followed by a digit, e.g., Yellow 5.

♦ For the most part, ingredients are given their scientific names. Prepare to see plenty of brain-boggling tongue-twisters. But there are occasions where they take up "common names", which feel a little more human, such as menthol instead of (1R, 2S, 5R)-2-isopropyl-5-methylcyclohexanol (thank goodness!). This is because they were already established names when the nomenclature system was set up. Botanical ingredients, such as essential oils and plant extracts, are mostly listed in Latin – good news only for classicists and keen gardeners, who will likely recognize a few.

Finding Out More About INCI Lists

In Europe brands have to display their INCIs, but in the US they often don't. If you're confused by any ingredient in your skincare product, there are three places you can go for further help:

1. The INCI dictionary: http://webdictionary. personalcarecouncil.org/ctfa-static/online/ FrontMatter_Vol1%20Edited%20for%20Websites. pdf

2. The brand itself. It's important to remember that most brands want to help. For the most part they are simply following legalities, as opposed to being purposely deceptive, by trying to squeeze an enormous amount of information onto a tiny label. If you ask them for further information, I think you'll be pleasantly surprised by the positive reaction you'll get back. There are a whole raft of product developers who work for brands that would be thrilled to know you are taking an interest in their work.

3. Google. The internet can do more harm than good, and is often a confusing place, but in the case of INCI listings it can be very helpful. In fact, there's a new trend for pasting INCI lists into a search engine and seeing what comes up: you can find reviews, debates, identical or near-identical products on the market, and so on.

4. Sometimes ingredients appear on the front of the label but actually constitute less than 1% in the

formula, which is why it's so important to check the INCI list. This is mismarketing at its worst, but it does happen. On the other hand, some brands won't list their percentages of ingredients at all, less to be deceptive and more because they worry about being duped.

Some things to remember about INCI lists:

♦ The scariest-sounding ingredients are often the kindest. Tocopherol? It's actually just a form of vitamin E. And salicylic acid, which sounds like something that might burn your skin, is an amazing cell-renewing ingredient that's brilliant for acne.

♦ "Chemical" doesn't necessarily mean "not natural". All substances in skincare are chemicals; it just means they're made from matter.

♦ Beware seven-digit codes. There's an INCI loophole whereby cosmetics companies can get away with not naming certain ingredients and instead listing a seven-digit code that means they don't need to declare the ingredient on the package.

♦ Don't lose heart at the sight of complex lists. It's getting increasingly easier to read them. As brands get used to the idea that their consumer might actually want to know the contents of their skincare, they are beginning to design labels that make the INCI list more accessible, providing explanations for scientific lingo and using bigger fonts. Cute naturals brand By Sarah is one example: it has begun to list all of the ingredients in layman's terms, in addition to the full scientific list on the back. Thank you, Sarah.

Deciphering INCI Lists

We have now arrived at the diagrams part of the book. This is the moment where you put into practice everything you have learned so far. All your time spent deciphering marketing terms and ingredient caveats will come into play when you're looking at product labels. Do the ingredients in the INCI list match up to what's mentioned on the front of the bottle? Are the quantities of the active ingredients high enough to be worth the money? Is the product going to work for your skin type? Are there any ingredients that you would now choose to avoid? This is your chance to take control of your skincare destiny.

In this section, I have provided you with the INCI listings for eight cult products. All the products are different, but, whether wholly natural, predominantly synthetic or a real mixture of the two, I have used them all and would use them again on my skin. I have selected the products not because I think they are the best or the worst, but because they give a good overview of what you might want to check when you start to do your own browsing.

It's important not to be intimidated when faced with an INCI list. You don't need to know the definition of every single chemical compound or scientific code. For the speedy mindful shopper, armed with knowledge from this book, there are certain clues to look out for. Within an INCI list you will find active ingredients (whether natural or synthetic; many naturals are indicated by their botanical names, or the word "extract" or "oil"), as well as "filler" ingredients that add texture and bulk, preservatives and stabilizers, colorants, fragrance, emollients (which make the skin feel softer), humectants (which add moisture), and emulsifiers and binders (which keep formulas together). You will soon be able to determine how concentrated a formula is, and the effect it might have on your skin.

A final note: ingredient lists do change – regularly, and for many reasons – so the labels you are about to see may well get updated, completely reformulated or simply tweaked for improvement at any time in the future.

WELEDA

Seit 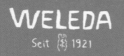 1921

Skin Food

Rich, Intensive
skin care

For very dry and rough skin

ORGANIC

 Certified Natural Skin Care

75 ml ℮

WELEDA

since 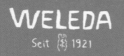 1921

Skin Food

Rich, intensive
skin care
For Face or Body
For very dry and rough skin

Certified Natural Skin Care

75 ml ℮

Case Study 1:
Weleda Skin Food

When Weleda says this is skin food, it's not far from the truth. Many of Weleda's ingredients are grown on their farms, using biodynamic farming methods (i.e. ultra-organic principles that are led by the natural climate and the cycles of the moon), so although they look fairly chemical as an INCI list, they are in fact 100% natural.

Water (Aqua) Used a lot in skincare because it's simple and rarely aggravates the skin. In hyper-natural products, it's predominantly used to create the right liquid consistency, and it's employed in the water/alcohol extraction process to draw out therapeutic plant actives from natural ingredients ♦ **Helianthus Annuus (Sunflower) Seed Oil** Contains antioxidant vitamin E, which helps to protect the skin from damage ♦ **Lanolin** Natural substance obtained from sheep's wool, used in formulas to protect skin ♦ **Prunus Amygdalus Dulcis** Not, in fact, prune but sweet almond oil, which is great for hydrating and softening – a super-ingredient to look out for if you have naturally dry or combination skin ♦ **Beeswax** Used to lock in moisture, creating a water-resistant barrier over the skin ♦ **Alcohol** Vodka? Tequila? Sadly not. In Weleda's case, it's an organic vegetable-based alcohol that's used in the extraction process to deliver all the goodness from the plant actives to the skin. When it comes to skincare, there are good alcohols and bad alcohols. The good alcohols – often prefixed by the words "cetyl", "stearyl" and "cetearyl" – are non-irritating. The bad ones – such as propyl alcohol – can be very drying on skin. You'll find the latter on the INCI list as "SD alcohol" or "Denatured alcohol". These can strip the skin of its good natural oils so shouldn't be used too frequently. Personally, I prefer my alcohol in a wine glass, but in this case it's harmless ♦ **Poly-glyceryl-3 Polyricinoleate** Emulsifier ♦ **Glycerin** Humectant ♦ **Limonene** A naturally occurring liquid that's part of the citrus family, this can help to make a product smell fresh and juicy. There is a synthetic version, but in Weleda's case, it's drawn from one of the aromatic essential oils that fragrances the product ♦ **Viola Tricolor Extract** Skin-soothing plant extract

♦ **Hydrolyzed Beeswax** Hydrolysis (sounds scary, it's not) is the process of turning something into liquid, often using an enzyme or acid. Here, natural beeswax is given a creamy consistency, and is then employed as an emulsifier and stabilizer, which thickens the texture of the formula and gives it that lovely balmy feel ♦ **Sorbitan Olivate** Fatty acids from olive oil mixed with a sugar called sorbitol, this is an emulsifier that is PEG-free and generally gentle on the skin ♦ **Rosmarinus Officinalis (Rosemary) Leaf Extract** A famous restorative and ingredient polymath: this invigorating ingredient can perk up a pasty complexion, and is a powerful antioxidant and antimicrobial ♦ **Chamomilla Recutita (Matricaria) Flower Extract** Skin-soothing extract from the camomile flower ♦ **Calendula Officinalis Flower Extract** From the pot marigold flower, included for its skin-healing anti-inflammatory and antibacterial properties ♦ **Arginine** Amino acid with antioxidant properties ♦ **Zinc Sulfate** Traditional, time-tested stabilizer, with handy antimicrobial properties ♦ **Fragrance (Parfum)** Fragrance, or parfum, can mask a multitude of sins. Many formulators use it to cover up slightly funky ingredient smells, while others add it for sensory effect. It's not compulsory for a brand to state whether their fragrance is natural or synthetically created. After a little digging on Weleda's website, you can rule out synthetic fragrances: in their case, it comes from essential oils only. This is good news, but not to be passed off as totally harmless, since essential oils can cause irritation to sensitive skin types and pregnant women ♦ **Linalool, Geraniol, Citral, Coumarin** Like Weleda's limonene, these are all naturally occurring compounds found in the pure essential oils that make up the classic scent of this product, including sweet orange and lavandulae.

Case Study 2:
Charlotte's Magic Cream

Is this cream really magic? It's certainly award-winning. Makeup artist Charlotte Tilbury was using this "secret-ingredient" cream on clients for years, stored in unbranded pots, before she bottled it (and disclosed her secret ingredient list) for her eponymous brand.

Water Used to combine formulas and help carry ingredients into the skin ◆ **Homosalate** UVB sunscreen ◆ **Glyceryl Stearate SE** Thickening agent (SE stands for self-emulsifying), helping to give the cream a luxurious richness ◆ **Ethylhexyl Salicylate** UVB sunscreen ◆ **Butylene Glycol** A common ingredient used to amplify texture. It's high up the INCI list, along with **Dimethicone** (a silicone used to give skin a smooth coating of product), meaning that the texture of the cream was high on the product developer's priority list ◆ **Glycerin** Humectant ◆ **Butyl Methoxydibenzoylmethane** Sunscreen (Paula's Choice website ranks this as one of the best) ◆ **Octocrylene** UVB sunscreen ◆ **Cetyl Alcohol** Non-irritating stabilizer ◆ **C12-15 Alkyl Benzoate** Emollient ◆ **Cyclopentasiloxane** A silicone (and therefore an emollient) ◆ **Phenoxyethanol** A widely used synthetic preservative ◆ **Butyrospermum Parkii** Nourishing shea butter ◆ **Steareth-21** Emulsifier ◆ **Avena Sativa (Oat) Kernel Extract** Antioxidant and anti-inflammatory ◆ **Carbomer** Emulsifier ◆ **Dimethiconol** A polymer similar to dimethicone (see above) ◆ **Potassium Cetyl Phosphate** Emulsifier ◆ **Chlorphenesin** Preservative ◆ **Caprylyl Glycol** Emollient (and sometimes preservative) ◆ **Xantham Gum** Incredibly common within skincare formulations; can either be an emulsifier or a thickening ingredient, giving that lovely rich texture ◆ **Hydrolyzed Viola Tricolor Extract** Skin-soothing pansy extract that has undergone a chemical process ◆ **Allantoin** Skin soother that can be found in nature (extracted from plants such as comfrey), but is most likely — for cost and convenience reasons — to be produced synthetically ◆ **Aloe Barbadensis Leaf Juice** Skin-soothing aloe vera ◆ **Disodium EDTA** Chelating agent, boosting preservation of the formula ◆ **Tocopheryl Acetate** Skin-repairing vitamin E ◆ **Camellia Oleifera Seed Oil** Natural plant oil ◆ **Rose Canina Fruit Oil** Natural plant oil, high in lovely fatty acids ◆ **Rosa Damascena Extract** Skin soother containing antioxidant properties ◆ **Sodium Hydroxide** Used to sustain the pH of a product; this might be one to avoid if you have very sensitive skin ◆ **Helianthus Annuus (Sunflower) Seed Oil** Contains antioxidant vitamin E, which helps to protect the skin from damage ◆ **Michelia Alba Leaf Oil** Natural essential oil ◆ **Sodium Lactate** May be used to sustain the pH of a product ◆ **Coco-glucoside** Cleansing agent ◆ **PEG-8** "PEG" stands for "polyethylene glycol" — a synthetic compound that's used for lots of different things in skincare because it's very versatile when mixed with other ingredients, is a good skin cleanser, and won't sting or irritate your eyes; here, it's used as a solvent and humectant ◆ **Ethylhexylglycerin** Preservative ◆ **Sodium Hyaluronate** A form of hyaluronic acid — very hydrating ◆ **Tocopherol** Vitamin E — quite far down on the INCI list, so it won't be in huge concentration, but it is an active ingredient ◆ **Palmitoyl Tetrapeptide-7, Palmitoyl Tripeptide-1** Anything ending in "peptide" is a good thing, indicating that a formula will have some rejuvenating effects on texture and structure of the skin ◆ **Ascorbyl Palmitate** Vitamin C ◆ **Plumeria Rubra Flower Extract** Used for natural fragrance ◆ **Ascorbic Acid** More vitamin C. Check for other antioxidants, as ascorbic acid works better when it has company. Here you've got **Citric acid** and a few others, which is good ◆ **Nicotiana Sylvestris Leaf Cell Culture** Skin conditioner ◆ **Linalool, Citronellol, Geraniol** All natural fragrances ◆ **Plus a little bit of top-secret "magic"** This is just (brilliant) marketing speak; a product has to be certified as legal for use in cosmetics by the EMA (Magic Cream's European ingredient list is given above) or the FDA in the US to get into the pot...

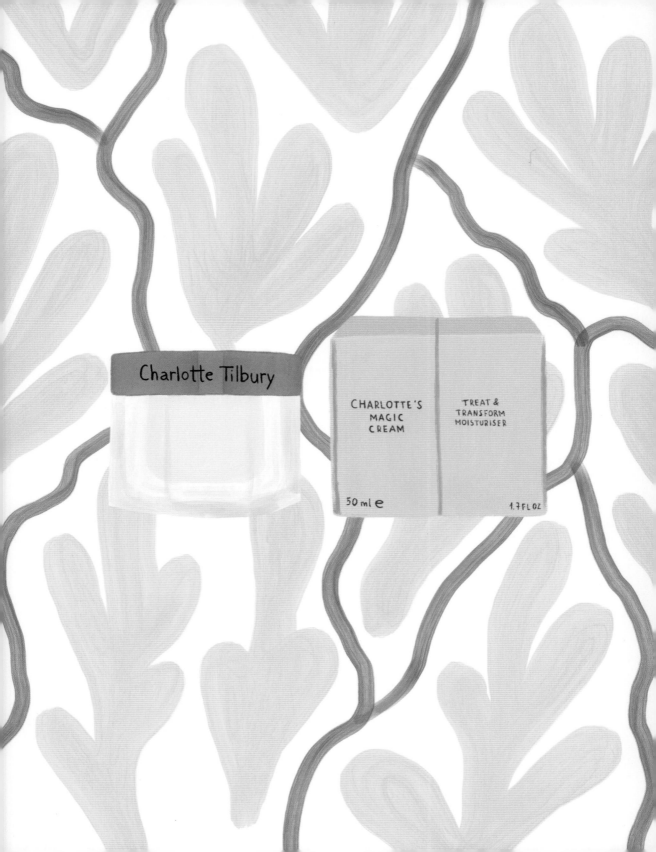

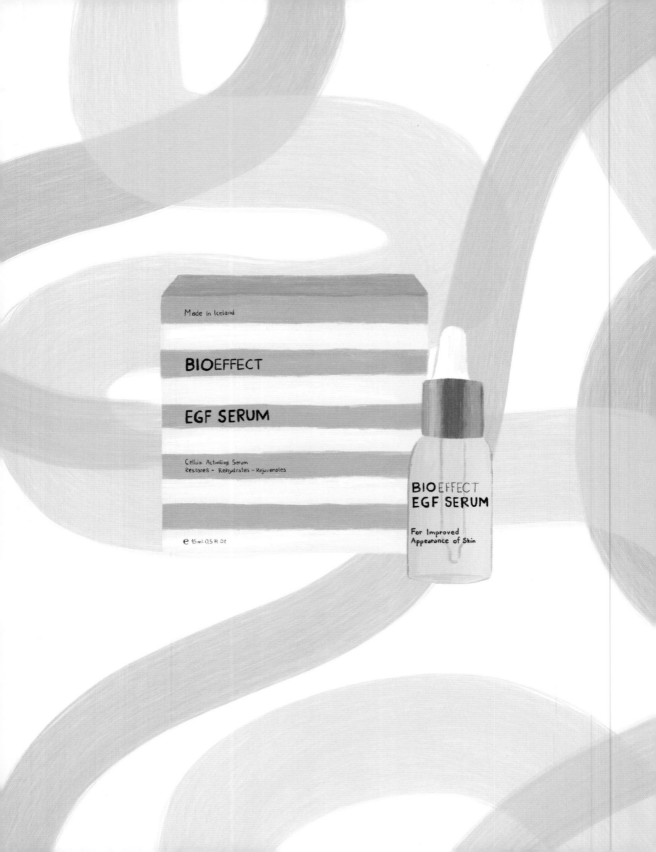

Case Study 3:
Bioeffect EGF Serum

One of the serums I really rate, both in terms of instant visible results and on account of the fact that it contains only seven ingredients! It is exceedingly rare in the skincare industry - even the beauty industry as a whole - for a product to have such a slimline INCI. Let's take a look at what it does contain.

Glycerin Glycerin is found in all sorts of cosmetics, from moisturizers to face masks, haircare and sunscreen. Its main purpose in a serum would likely be to attract moisture to the skin and hold it there for a smoother surface texture. It's a naturally occurring compound that can be derived from both plants and animals, and it can be produced synthetically. Having it frontloaded as it is on this INCI list means that you can expect a glow soon after applying ◆ **Water (Aqua)** After a little digging on the Bioeffect website, we discover that this is in fact Icelandic water, which we know is much softer than other waters and therefore gentler on the skin. If you've ever swum in the blue lagoon outside of Reykjavik, you will have felt the benefits of Icelandic water first-hand ◆ **Sodium Hyaluronate** Another name for hyaluronic acid, which is a naturally occurring molecule famous for holding up to 1,000 times its own weight in water. In short, it is the don of all moisturizers ◆ **Tromethamine** Used in cosmetics as a pH adjustor. Why would you want to adjust the pH of your skincare? Some ingredients and preservatives need to remain at a certain pH in order to function efficaciously ◆ **Sodium Chloride** Salt, used to control the viscosity of a product ◆ **Barley (Hordeum Vulgare) Seed Extract** Barley seed extract does contain some antioxidant properties, but Bioeffect use it as a foundation on which to grow their bioengineered replica of human growth factor EGF. The barley is grown in beds of Icelandic pumice granules in a carbon-neutral greenhouse in Iceland. I've been there — it's amazing, and about as wholesome as science comes ◆ **EGF (Barley SH-Oligopeptide-1)** This is a plant-based replica of a human (epidermal) growth factor which, when applied topically, encourages your skin cells to power up, increasing turnover whilst boosting production of collagen and elastin. The fact that this growth factor is grown on a crop of plants is particularly important, since many growth factors in cosmetics are produced on bacteria or even human cells, which of course raises a few ethical alarm bells.

Case Study 4:
Glossier Solution

Dubbed the answer to dull skin woes, Glossier Solution got some rave reviews when it launched. It's a skin-resurfacing tonic, designed to give you a fresher appearance.

Water Used to combine formulas and help carry ingredients into the skin ◆ **Acids** There are lots of acids listed in Solution – from **Lactic** and **Glycolic** to **Citric** and **Acetic**. This is less scary than it sounds, and means that the product has an emphasis on chemical exfoliation, helping to lift off dead skin from the surface and provide a smoother, brighter-looking complexion ◆ **Gluconolactone** The hero ingredient in this product (NB in the US version, the main ingredient is salicylic acid; see further on in this INCI list). Gluconolactone is a PHA (a polyhydroxy acid) and one of the gentlest on the market, while still being pretty effective. It can be used daily, and can also be used by people with sensitive skin ◆ **Propanediol** Enhances the absorption of other ingredients in the formula. Propanediol can be natural, or can be synthetic, depending on an individual brand's needs ◆ **Aloe Barbadensis Leaf Juice** Skin-soothing aloe vera ◆ **Ethoxydiglycol** Solvent used to thin out the formula ◆ **Magnesium Chloride** Thickening agent ◆ **Sodium Hydroxide** Used to sustain the pH of a product; this might be one to avoid if you have very sensitive skin ◆ **Glycereth-7 Trimethyl Ether** Emollient ◆ **Niacinamide** Vitamin B3, which helps to reduce the appearance of enlarged pores and hyperpigmentation – a great active ingredient that should be included in your regime ◆ **Betaine** Hydrating ingredient (again, this can be natural or synthetic, depending on the product) ◆ **Inositol**, **Glycerin** Humectants ◆ **Salicylic Acid** Another of Solution's chemical exfoliators, helping to unclog pores and lift off dead skin. It's great for blemish-prone skin ◆ **Phytic Acid** An AHA (alpha hydroxy acid), helping to peel away dead skin from the surface ◆ **Pentylene Glycol** Humectant ◆ **PEG-60 Hydrogenated Castor Oil** Emollient ◆ **Caprylyl Glycol** Emollient, and sometimes preservative (as an ingredient, it can be natural or synthetic) ◆ **Ethylhexylglycerin** Preservative ◆ **Fragrance** Again, depending on a particular brand/product, fragrance can be natural or synthetic ◆ **PEG-8** PEG (polyethylene glycol) is very versatile when mixed with other ingredients, and is a good skin cleanser ◆ **Potassium Hydroxide** Sustains the pH of a product.

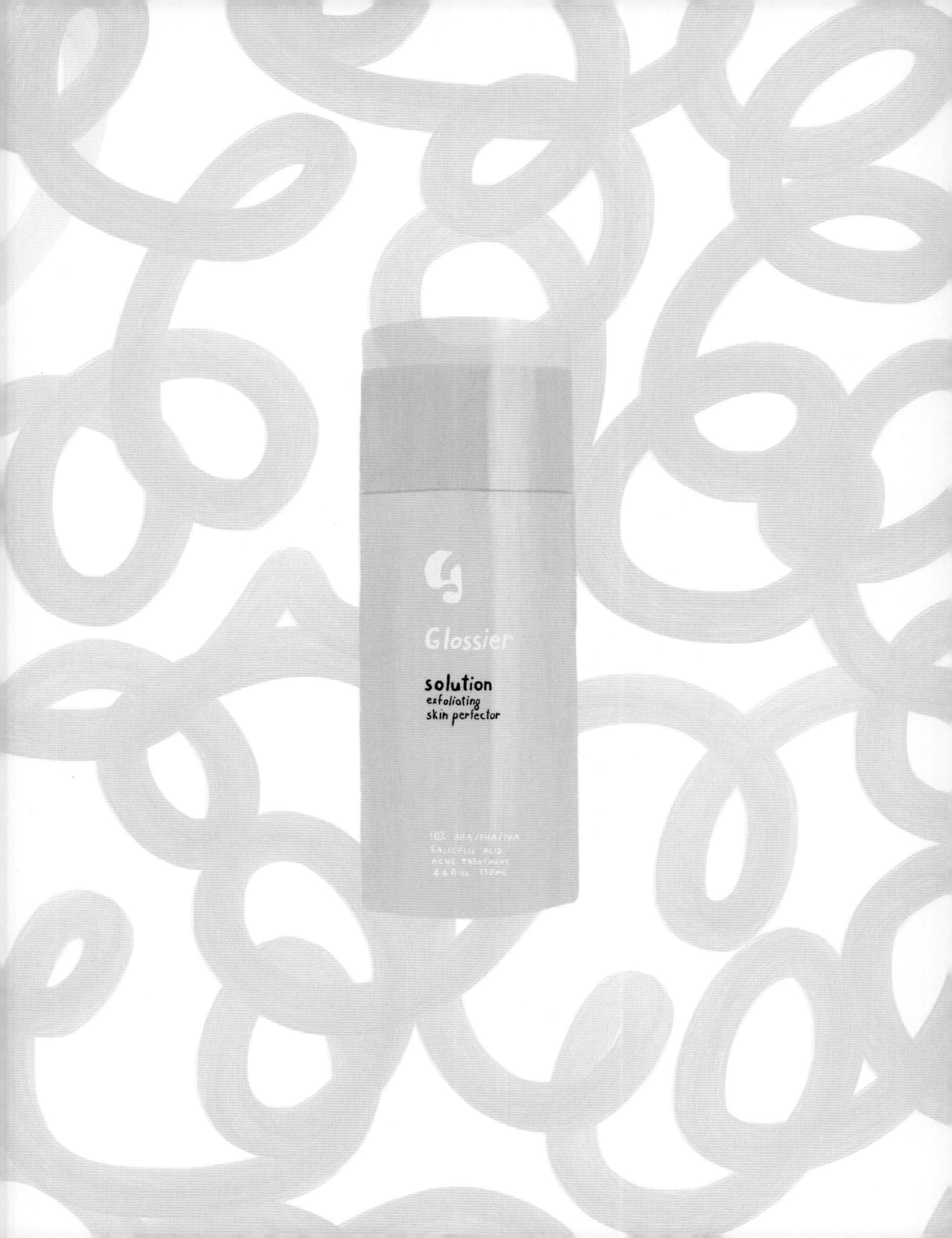
Glossier
solution
exfoliating
skin perfector
SALICYLIC ACID
ACNE TREATMENT

thisworks

24 HR SKIN SOLUTIONS

morning expert™ hyaluronic serum

2% Hyaluronic Acid & slow release Vitamin C help plump & brighten morning skin

sérum repulpant visage et cou à l'acide hyaluronique

30 ml ℮ 1 fl oz

---

morning expert™ hyaluronic serum

2% Hyaluronic Acid & slow release Vitamin C help plump & brighten morning skin

sérum repulpant visage et cou à l'acide hyaluronique

thisworks®

30 ml ℮ 1 fl oz

Case Study 5:
This Works Morning Expert Hyaluronic Serum

This Works' products are categorized by the optimum time of day for using them - a smart way of organizing your regime, especially since we know that your skin needs different things round the clock. Their Morning Expert range contains specific ingredients that rehydrate skin on waking, energizing and protecting it for the day ahead. Let's take a look at what these are:

Aqua (Water) Used to combine formulas and help carry ingredients into the skin ◆ **Glycerin** A humectant ◆ **Ascorbyl Glucoside** This is a form of Vitamin C, which is an antioxidant, great for brightening and evening skin tone, but also a good thing to load your skin with at the start of a busy day, as it will help protect skin from free radical damage brought on by environmental aggressors such as pollution ◆ **Sodium Hyaluronate** Another name for hyaluronic acid, a top-notch moisturizing molecule that is naturally found in skin and can hold up to 1,000 times its own weight in water. Finding it this high up the ingredient list is a good sign, because our skin loses a lot of moisture overnight and needs topping up in the morning in order to restore its fresh appearance ◆ **Albizia Julibrissin (Persian Silk Tree) Bark Extract** The Persian silk tree is a small south-east Asian tree with a stripy bark and a bright pink blossom. You'll find it used in brightening or anti-skin-fatigue formulations because it's an active anti-glycation ingredient, meaning it helps to support the skin's natural detoxification processes and stops the breakdown of proteins like collagen in your skin ◆ **Heptyl Glucoside** This helps the active ingredients in the formula better penetrate the skin ◆ **PEG-40 Hydrogenated Castor Oil** An emollient ◆ **Phenoxyethanol** A commonly used synthetic preservative: Paula's Choice ingredient dictionary rates it as a 'good' ingredient. It's approved for safe use in skincare at a concentration of 1% but, as with many synthetic preservatives, it receives some negative attention online ◆ **Sodium Levulinate** This helps to condition and soften the skin ◆ **Benzyl Alcohol** A great anti-microbial ingredient, which means it's a good choice for those who have blemishes or suffer from acne ◆ **Marrubium Vulgare (Horehound) Extract** A soothing natural ingredient that is good at reducing redness – perfect for those who wake up a bit red or blotchy ◆ **Sodium Anisate** A natural preservative found in fennel ◆ **Xanthan Gum** A sugar that is very common within skincare formulations, and can either be an emulsifier or a thickening ingredient ◆ **Sodium Hydroxide** Used to balance the pH of a product to ensure compatibility with the skin ◆ **Phytic Acid** An antioxidant ◆ **Ethylhexylglycerin** A synthetic preservative ◆ **Parfum (Fragrance)** We know from This Works' website that they never use synthetic fragrances or perfumes; they only use high-grade essential oils to scent their products ◆ **Dehydroacetic Acid** A synthetic preservative ◆ **Linalool** Fragrance ingredient ◆ **Heptanol** Also a fragrance ingredient ◆ **Sodium Benzoate** A synthetic preservative made from benzoic acid, which can be found naturally in some fruit; Paula's Choice ingredient dictionary rates it as a 'good' ingredient ◆ **Citric Acid** A natural extract that can help adjust the pH of a formula; as an AHA, in the right product and concentration it can also promote skin exfoliation ◆ **Limonene** A natural citrus fragrance.

Case Study 6:
Chanel La Crème Main

These pebble-shaped pots are possibly the chicest packaging I've ever seen, and have an equally sophisticated-looking ingredient list. Let's see what the INCI list tells us.

Water Used to combine formulas and help carry ingredients into the skin ♦ **Glycerin** Humectant ♦ **C13–16 Isoparaffin** Petroleum-derived texture enhancer ♦ **Dimethicone** Synthetic silicone used to provide slip, leaving skin with a smooth coating of product ♦ **Cetyl Alcohol** Non-irritating stabilizer ♦ **Pentylene Glycol** Humectant ♦ **Jojoba Esters** These are the hydrogenation product of jojoba (pronounced "ho-ho-ba") oil. Jojoba is a great moisturizer, containing a mix of vitamins A, E and D, plus antioxidants and fatty acids, and is used in a wide variety of beauty products ♦ **Glyceryl Stearate** Emollient ♦ **Acacia Decurrens Flower Wax** Skin-protecting natural wax, from the mimosa flower ♦ **Rosa Centifolia Flower Wax** Rosa centifolia is the beautifully scented Rose de Mai, which is grown in fields exclusively for Chanel in Grasse, the south of France. I have seen it harvested, distilled and bottled with my own eyes. You don't get more natural than this. In wax form, it will help to protect and nourish the skin, keeping moisture locked in ♦ **Iris Pallida Root Extract** Iris essential oil brightens, tightens and firms skin ♦ **Glycyrrhiza Glabra** Liquorice root extract is a great natural ingredient for super-dry skin – excellent on cracked heels and stubborn dry patches like shins and elbows, too ♦ **Panthenol** Hydrating vitamin B5 ♦ **Polyglycerin-3** Humectant ♦ **Ethyl Oleate** Emollient ♦ **PEG-75 Stearate** Emulsifier ♦ **Phenoxyethanol** Synthetic preservative ♦ **Silica** Thickener, emulsifier ♦ **Tocopheryl Acetate** Antioxidant vitamin E ♦ **Propanediol** Enhances the absorption of other ingredients in the formula – can be natural, can be synthetic ♦ **Butylene Glycol** A common ingredient used in cream to amplify the texture ♦ **Ethyl Stearate** Skin smoother ♦ **Chlorphenesin** Synthetic preservative ♦ **Caprylyl Glycol** Emollient, and sometimes preservative (can be natural or synthetic) ♦ **Dimethicone** Synthetic silicone used to provide slip, leaving skin with a smooth coating of product ♦ **Sodium Carbomer** Helps stabilize the formula ♦ **Ceteth-20** Emollient ♦ **Steareth-20** Emulsifier ♦ **Xantham Gum** A sugar that is very common within skincare formulations, and can either be an emulsifier or a thickening ingredient ♦ **Parfum** Note that fragrance isn't listed at the end of the INCI, indicating that the product is going to smell of perfume quite noticeably. Could be a good thing, could be a bad thing, depending on how/whether you like your skincare scented ♦ **Butyrospermum Parkii (Shea Butter)** Anti-inflammatory, healing, soothing skin softener ♦ **Ethyl Linoleate** Antibacterial, anti-inflammatory fatty acid ♦ **Helianthus Annuus Seed Wax** Natural thickener and emulsifier ♦ **Caprylic/Capric Triglyceride** Emollient ♦ **Sodium Hyaluronate** A form of hyaluronic acid – very hydrating ♦ **Sodium Citrate** Controls the pH of the formula ♦ **Phytic Acid** A natural AHA ♦ **Citric Acid** A fruit extract that can help adjust the pH of a formula; as an AHA, in the right product and concentration it can also promote skin exfoliation ♦ **Tocopherol** Another form of vitamin E ♦ **Sodium Benzoate** A fruit-derived preservative.

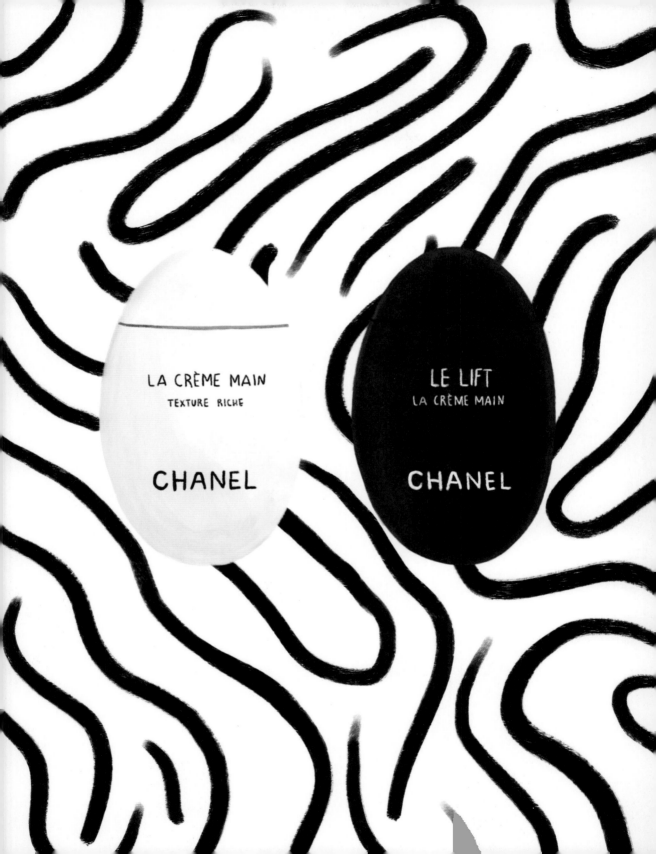

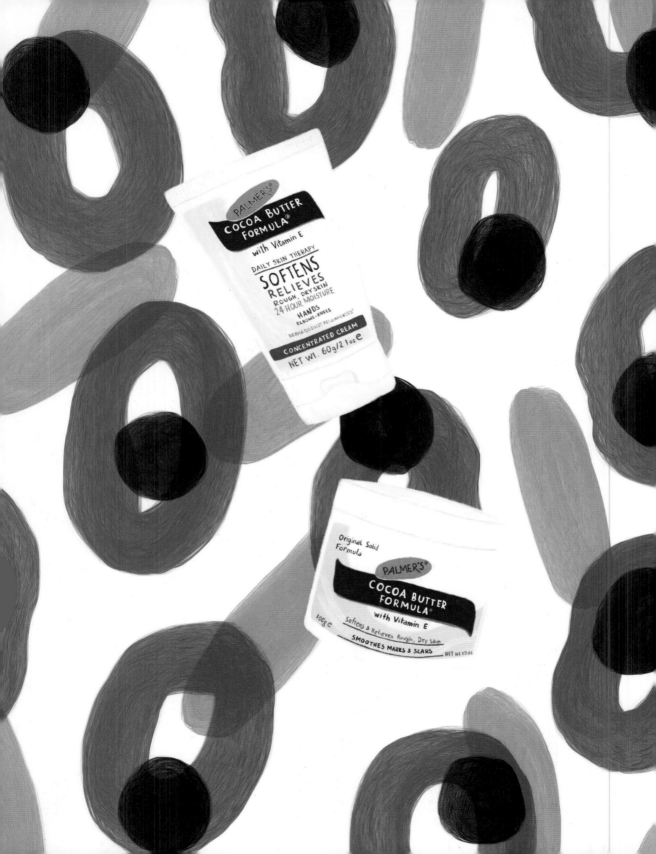

Case Study 7:
Palmer's Cocoa Butter Formula

A high-street hero and a number one holiday pack for many. Does this wallet-friendly wonder do wonders for your skin? I've certainly always been coco-nuts for its Piña Colada scent. Here's the INCI list for Palmer's jar of Original Solid Formula.

Theobroma Cacao Extract This cocoa extract relieves dryness and reduces moisture loss, helping to keep skin hydrated for longer (Palmer's attest that the jar has been tested clinically to prove that it's effective for hydrating and moisturizing skin, and is suitable for eczema-prone skin, too) ♦ **Paraffinum Liquidum** Mineral oil, helping the skin to retain moisture; it's a petroleum by-product, however, which some may prefer to avoid ♦ **Cera Microcristallina** This highly refined microcrystalline wax is also derived from petroleum; it's used as a thickener and gives a nice, smooth, solid/semi-solid texture ♦ **Theobroma Cacao Seed Butter** Cocoa butter, a healing emollient, which Palmer's source ethically and sustainably from Ghana ♦ **Dimethicone** Synthetic silicone used to provide slip, leaving skin with a smooth coating of product ♦ **Parfum** For the price point you can place a fairly safe bet that this moisturizer is fragranced synthetically ♦ **Tocopheryl** Natural antioxidant vitamin E, helping to protect the skin from damage ♦ **Helianthus Annuus Seed Oil** Another natural form of vitamin E ♦ **Beta Carotene (CI 40800)** Colorant ♦ **Zea Mays (Corn) Oil** Emollient ♦ **Isopropyl Myristate** Emollient, which can also help thicken formulations for a denser, more luxurious texture ♦ **Benzyl Benzoate** Widely used in skincare products, mainly as a fragrance ingredient ♦ **Benzyl Cinnamate** Fragrance ingredient.

Case Study 8:
Lush Honey Lip Scrub

A humble lip scrub, but a makeup artist staple.
Why? The INCI list is filled with promising-sounding
natural ingredients, and only ten of them, which is
refreshingly minimal for a cosmetic, but how does that
add up for your lips?

Caster Sugar Far superior to plastic microbeads, sugar granules make for a great physical scrub that won't pollute the oceans, and you can feel confident it won't harm you either if you accidentally swallow a bit ◆ **Organic Jojoba Oil** Jojoba is an ingredient that is universally used in a wide variety of beauty products, from the extremely expensive to the cheap and cheerful. It's a great moisturizer and contains a mix of vitamins A, E and D, plus antioxidants and fatty acids. It's also been credited with helping to prevent cold sores from forming, so is a great ingredient in a lip scrub. The Lush website lists their oil as coming from a sustainable producer in Peru ◆ **Vegan White Chocolate** There are antioxidant properties in cocoa, but the informal language makes it hard to tell whether this is melted Milkybar or something more wholesome. It's definitely vegan, though, which is a plus now for many consumers

◆ **Flavor (Fragrance)** A term used to describe an ingredient or group of ingredients that give both taste and scent to a cosmetic ◆ **Peppermint Oil** NB This can be skin-sensitizing ◆ **Vanilla Absolute** According to the Lush website, the vanilla pods used are Fairtrade from Madagascar. Personally, I love the scent of vanilla – although the quality of the ingredient can make the sophistication of the scent vary dramatically ◆ **Sweet Wild Orange Oil** An uplifting, bright scent in aromatherapy ◆ **Honey** There's a reason why honey has been used in natural beauty for millennia, including by the Ancient Greeks and Egyptians. It's antimicrobial, antifungal, moisturizing (it's a natural humectant) and, of course, it smells delicious ◆ **Alpha-isomethyl Ionone** Another fragrance and taste/flavour ingredient (this one's synthetic); avoid if you have sensitive skin ◆ **Limonene** Citrus fragrance.

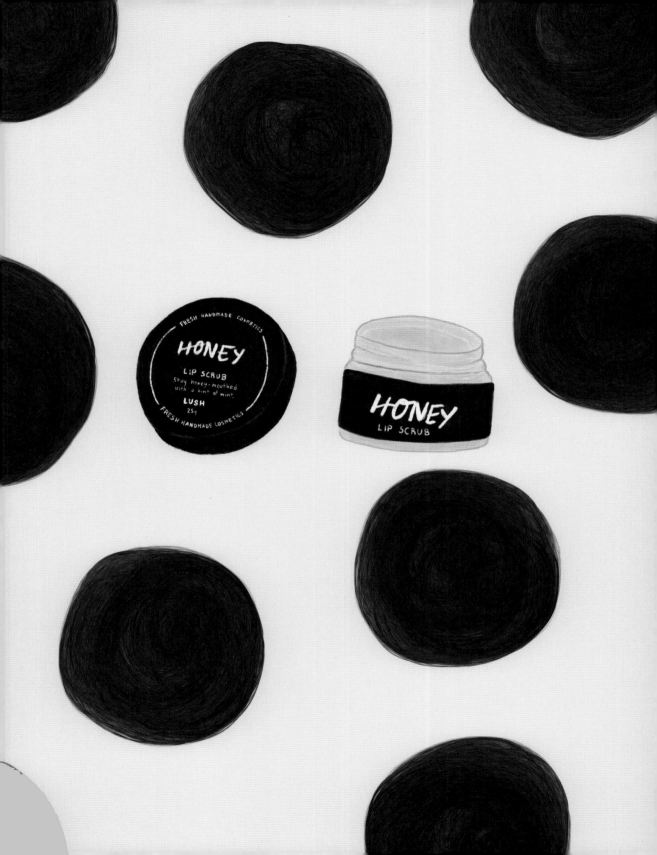

Tips and Notes

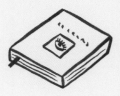

Diarize your Skincare

Once/twice a week: Do an at-home overnight peel once a week if you have sensitive skin or are trying peels for the first time. When you're sure your skin is used to it, you can try two times a week, but once is enough for my skin. Check the percentage and type of acid, as this will also dictate how often you should be using it.

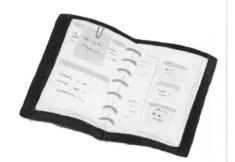

Twice a month/once a week: Do an LED facial either twice a month or once a week if you have blemish-prone skin.

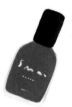

Every three weeks: I do a pedicure once every three weeks. I also thoroughly recommend having a medical pedicure once a year; it will make your pedicures last longer.

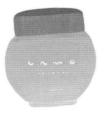

Once a month: I like to have a regular facial once a month – almost like a skin MOT. Depending on where my skin is at that month I will opt for a relaxing facial or a more functional one.

Every six months: My recommendation if you are going to have Botox is every six months. It gives you a little breathing space to live with your wrinkles again before you have your next treatment. You may decide you like them after all!

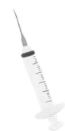

Twice a year: Try a hammam before a beach holiday. A hammam will do wonders for exfoliating and smoothing the look of the rough skin that builds up over the year.

Global Beauty Hotspots

You've read all about K-Beauty and French pharmacies (more below), but there are plenty of other skincare regions worth knowing about.

Australia: Home of a plethora of natural brands including Kora Organics, Alpha-H and Becca, among other brands.

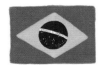

Brazil: Brazil is considered a hotspot for aesthetic body treatments and attracts plenty of tourism trade. Its skincare market has also picked up pace recently, with products such as Brazilian Bum Bum Cream becoming global cult bodycare buys.

France: There is something eternally covetable about chic French pharmacy brands and their white functional bottles. Look out for Klorane (which does a great dry shampoo), Bioderma (famous for its micellar water) and backstage makeup artist favourite Embryolisse Crème, which I have recommended to people with sensitive skin many times – even women who are undergoing chemotherapy.

Germany: Known for its groundbreaking dermatologist brands such as Dr Barbara Sturm, Augustinus Bader, Weleda and Dr Hauschka.

Iceland: It may be a small island but definitely don't overlook Iceland as a producer of great beauty brands. Bioeffect and Skyn Iceland (the latter is actually a British brand, but uses Icelandic ingredients) are two of my favourites.

Japan: Clé de Peau, Sensai, Shiseido – there are too many good skincare brands from Tokyo to mention. The Japanese place heavy importance on research, excellence and design, which make for an impressive combination when it comes to beauty products. One to pick out from the crowd is UKA, which creates beautiful scalp oils and an incredible scalp massage tool that I use every time I wash my hair.

South Korea: Home of sheet masks, snail slime, egg white foams and konjac sponges.

USA: Booming with exciting brands such as Drunk Elephant, CeraVe, Tata Harper and Vintner's Daughter.

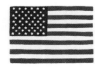

My Favourite Facial Destinations

The De Mamiel Urban Warrior facial

The Ned

The De Mamiel Urban Warrior facial at The Ned, London. Therapeutic, calming and luxurious. The facial is designed to unlock tension held in the face. I challenge you not to fall asleep.

Decorte Signature Infusion Ritual

Harrods

Using the Japanese brand's incredible AQ Meliority products, this facial is all about deep moisturization and cleansing but comes with a killer "onjun" head and décolleté massage. I've tried it in Tokyo and I've tried it in London – it never fails to be the most utterly blissful experience.

The Runway facial

The New York Dermatology Group

The Runway facial at the New York Dermatology Group, 5th Avenue, New York. Functional and fast, but packs a lot in, including LED, radiofrequency, dermabrasion and a peel. You can also find this at Harrods in London.

Teresa Tarmey's Townhouse

Teresa Tarmey's Townhouse, London. A decadent interiors heaven and A-list hangout, but the most hi-tech, hard-working facial experience I've had. You'll get extraction, too, and your face will feel squeakier than squeaky clean afterwards.

The Darphin Institute

The Darphin Institute, Place Vendôme, Paris. Darphin's balms, masks and creams are exquisitely sensorial when used at home, but when applied by the Institute you'll be sent to skincare cloud 9.

Skincare Treatment

Light Salon

Not technically a full facial, but I recommend the skincare treatment at the Light Salon, London, to anyone who is suffering from dull skin or skin that is prone to breakouts. Sitting under the LED lamp is an uplifting experience in itself, and you'll leave the chair looking and feeling much better.

How to Build a Basic Skincare Regime

Divide your day up into the number of times you would like to be applying skincare (a minimum of two if you can – morning and evening). Some people like to do a freshen-up around lunch, or after work, or after a gym session. I even like to have a mini-regime for my desk, but I am an extreme case...

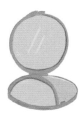

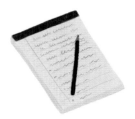

Spend a couple of days assessing your skin at different times of the day, taking notes on how it feels to the touch and how it looks. It might, for example, be super-dry and dull in the morning but red and greasy by 3pm (most people do wake up with dehydrated skin, and sebum levels naturally do increase over the course of the day). Also, remember that sometimes excessively oily skin can be a result of your skin actually being dehydrated. Think about what your skin might need in different time phases.

Build a skin wardrobe of just six simple products, and use them at times that match your unique skin diary. These should cover: a moisturizer, an antioxidant serum, a cleanser, a makeup remover or deep cleanser (these are not necessarily the same thing, since in the morning you don't need to remove makeup or pollution/grime from your skin with your cleanser), an SPF, and a primer or luminizer (I always recommend a luminizer as it makes such a difference to the look of your skin, whether you wear foundation or not).

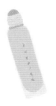

Test these out for a couple of weeks and discover where your gaps are. Are your lips feeling dry, for example? Time to add a lip oil. Do you find a double cleanse still leaves your pores feeling clogged? Time to try a chemical exfoliator or scrub. Are you finding your skin texture is still making you look tired? Time to look for some skin-lifting actives to add into your serum stage.

Figure out your skin tone using the Fitzpatrick chart overleaf. This defines your photo-sensitivity, and means you can make informed decisions about the SPF you should use and how often to reapply.

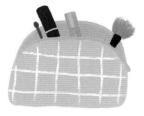

Have patience. Building your own skincare regime takes time. It should be fun as well, so enjoy mixing things up and trying new products if you feel the last one wasn't doing its job properly, until you find a regime that feels effortless and gives you glowy skin that people comment on.

How do I know my skin tone?

The Fitzpatrick scale is a measurement system for skin tone devised in 1975 and is used by most derms. Although there are infinite shades of skin, the Fitzpatrick scale is able to place them all under six categories, and it classifies skin type according to the amount of pigmentation in your skin. Where Type 1 is extremely fair in colour and burns easily, Type 6 is extremely dark and never freckles or burns. Fun fact: you may be amused to discover that the Fitzpatrick scale is what the skin tones of emojis are based upon. Check out where you sit on the spectrum below.

Type I -

always burns,
never tans
(palest; freckles)

Type II -

usually burns,
tans minimally

Type III -

sometimes burns
mildly, tans
uniformly

Type IV -

burns minimally,
always tans well
(moderate brown)

Type V -

very rarely burns,
tans very easily
(dark brown)

Type VI -

never burns
(deeply pigmented
dark brown to
darkest brown)

Notes

Armed with this "skinformation" and your newly formed skincare regime, you are now ready to go out and make some smart beauty purchases. It's time to sort through your bathroom #shelfie, make some lists on the notes pages that follow, and review your skincare routines (pp. 78, 86, 114 and 124). You'll be glowing in no time.

Notes

Notes

Notes

Notes

Notes

Further Reading

Here are my favourite websites and books for further reading on skincare and ingredients:

Alessandra Steinherr, https://www.instagram.com/alexsteinherr: Check out Alessandra Steinherr's Sunday Night Facial on Instagram. This ex-*Glamour* beauty director has a skincare regime to die for and incredible skin to show for it. Every Sunday she reveals her pampering process and it's extremely insightful.

Ask Mira, https://www.askmira.com: This search engine website has launched with the aim of being the Google for beauty products.

British Association of Aesthetic Plastic Surgeons, https://baaps.org.uk: The website for the British Association of Aesthetic Plastic Surgeons is great for the latest updates and press releases in the plastic surgery and injectables world.

Caroline Hirons, www.carolinehirons.com: Facialist and beauty influencer Caroline Hirons has reviewed all the latest skincare launches and is always honest in her write-up. An essential read before you buy, along with her book *skinCARE*.

The Essence of Perfume, perfume master Roja Dove's book, is my fragrance ingredient bible. Although it's not technically about skincare, many of the ingredients such as essential oils cross over, and it's a fascinating read.

Lisa Eldridge, www.lisaeldridge.com: This site is predominantly for makeup, but Lisa Eldridge often gives great skincare shopping advice. She uses a huge amount of skincare in her job and so is a real authority.

Lush, https://uk.lush.com: I often find myself on this site, reading up on natural ingredients.

Paula Begoun, www.paulaschoice.com, aka the Cosmetics Cop, is the original skincare sleuth from the pre-beauty-blogging days. Her website has an amazing glossary of skincare ingredients that is factual and clinical study-led.

Palette, Funmi Fetto's book, is an encyclopaedia of beauty product recommendations for women of colour. A must read.

Acknowledgments

This book could not have been written without the amazing insights of the following beauty experts: Florence Adepoju, Dr Yannis Alexandrides, Victoria Buchanan, Mia Collins, Olivia de Courcy, Shabir Daya, Roja Dove, George Driver, Montasar Dumas, Funmi Fetto, Haley Bloom Fitzpatrick, Lisa Goldfaden, Dr David Jack, Ateh Jewel, Nichola Joss, Sarah Jossel, Millie Kendall, Hannah Martin, Dr Björn Örvar, Kathy Phillips, Annabel Rivkin, Morag Ross, Teresa Tarmey, Zoë Taylor and Charlotte Tilbury. Thanks, too, to George Driver for research assistance.

Thank you to my sister Louisa and mother Amanda for reading endless drafts, and my beautiful daughter Aurelia for falling asleep in her pram enough for me to write this.

To all the strong women in my life, from Emma and Kathy to Kay, Olivia, Ella, Cassandra, and of course Emily (who is more obsessed with skincare than me): I love you all, this is for you.

About the Author

Katie Service is a beauty editor, whose first job within the industry was as a makeup artist, working for beauty legends Kay Montano, Charlotte Tilbury and Alex Box. As a journalist, she has held posts at *Sunday Times Style*, *InStyle* and *ES Magazine*, as well as writing for titles such as *ID* online, *ALSO Journal*, *Vogue* China, *Vogue* Japan and *LFW Daily*. She is also the co-founder of her own beauty creative agency, Runway Beauty, and is one of the four founding partners of beauty community, The Beauty Conversation.

A regular backstage reporter at London, Paris, Milan and New York fashion weeks, Katie works with some of the industry's top creatives, from photographers such as Jem Mitchell and Jason Hetherington to makeup artists and hairstylists such as Lisa Eldridge, Andrew Gallimore and Sam McKnight, as well as brands including Chanel, Tom Ford and This Works.

Katie lives in London with her husband Aaron and daughter Aurelia, and is currently beauty editorial director at Harrods.

Index

Main entries are indicated in **bold**

Tilbury, Charlotte 9, 55, 142, 172,
titanium dioxide 93, 94, **95**
tocopherol *see* vitamin E
Tom Ford Beauty 65
toner 31, 42, 45, 71, **104**, 115
toothpaste (on spots) 130, **131**
touch therapy 148, **149**
transepidermal water loss (TEWL) 54, 57, **104**
travel minis **84**
travelling skin care 83–7, 90, 103, 30, 45, 71, 76
tretinoin *see* retinoic acid
triclocarbon **91**
triclosan **91**, 130, 131
turmeric **39**, 57, 119, 127
Typology (cosmetics) 164

ubiquinone *see* coenzyme Q10
UKA 191
ultherapy **150**
ultrasound facials **150**
undereye bags 119
United States Department of Agriculture (USDA) 167
urban acne 18
USA 191
use-by dates **24–5**, 166
UVA light **95**
UVB light **95**, 172

vagus nerve 99
Valnet, Jean 31
Vaseline (cosmetics) 91
vegan skincare 7, 11, **14–15**, 17, 30, 76, 89, 112, 157, 167, 184
velvet 17, **62**
vitamin A 15, **112**, 129, 149
    see also retinol
vitamin C 30, 34, **39**, 45, 53, 57, 79, 95, 97, 107, 144, 172, 179
vitamin E 25, 33, **39**, 47, 84, 107, 121, 169, 171, 172, 180, 183
Votary (cosmetics) 13

water
    in the body 91
    carbonated 74
    cold 99, 105
    hot water 104, 105
    ice **121**
    Icelandic 33
    loss 91
    salt 129
    sources **108**
        see also aqua
water-based cleansers 45, 71, **77**
water-based ingredients 33, 38, 41, 42, **57**
water-based products 25, 42, 57, 61, 98
WaterAid (organization) 11
Weleda Skin Food **171**
white light facials 144, **150**
        see also LED light facials
whitening *see* skin lightening

YAG Laser (cosmetic procedure) **150**

Zelens (cosmetics) 45
zinc oxide 93, 94, **95**, 121, 127, 131

First published in the United Kingdom in 2021
by Thames & Hudson Ltd, 181A High Holborn,
London WC1V 7QX

First published in the United States of America
in 2021 by Thames & Hudson Inc., 500 Fifth
Avenue, New York, New York 10110

British Library Cataloguing-in-Publication Data
A catalogue record for this book is available from
the British Library

Library of Congress Control Number 2020931830

ISBN 978-0-500-29546-5

Printed and bound in China by C & C Offset Printing Co. Ltd

Be the first to know about our new releases,
exclusive content and author events by visiting
thamesandhudson.com
thamesandhudsonusa.com
thamesandhudson.com.au